Man Against Mortality

Man Against Mortality

or

'Seven Essays on the Engineering of Man's Divinity'

D. F. Juniper

Charles Scribner's Sons
New York

1 3 5 7 9 11 13 15 17 19 I/C 20 18 16 14 12 10 8 6 4 2

Printed in Great Britain
Library of Congress Catalog Card Number 74-4814
ISBN 0-684-13884-0

Preface

This book is an attempt to analyse seven views of man freed from the restraints of immortality. In this regard it is closely linked with modern theological thinking which has come to view man as a kind of demi-God. Although none of the essays attempts any absolute definition of mortality, it is necessary to make some attempt at this early point. For our present purposes, immortality is operationally defined as the amount of time that any man might wish to live supposing that he had the power to do so. This is an open-ended definition and immortality is thus presented as a state of absolute choice which must, of course, be underpinned by the kinds of absolute refinements of technology which allow continuous life to become feasible.

The first essay discusses attitudes in relation to this kind of absolute choice, together with the restrictions of extended lifespans. We move on from this to consider the surgical, biological, engineering, cybernetic and sociological impacts of extended lifespans, and end with an examination of the nature of immortality as it might be experienced psychologically.

Acknowledgements

Acknowledgements are dangerous for two reasons. First, those who are acknowledged may not wish to be associated with the results of their assistance, while those who are omitted may paradoxically feel slighted. I apologize in advance for both these possibilities. Nevertheless, I most gratefully acknowledge the following people in various fields, without whose help this book could not have been completed. I am linking them with the chapters to which they principally contributed:

Current Views. Rev. Denys Whiteley, Jesus College, Oxford; The late Mr. Roy Neate; Dr. J. Thompson, Easthampstead Park College; Professor Ray Wilson, School of Education, Reading University.

Not All Their Own. Miss Mary Tisserand, *Bio-medical Engineering;* Dr. John Martin, Atomic Weapons Research Establishment; Mr. David Fishlock, *Financial Times*; Mr. S. J. Charters, School of Education, Reading University.

The Engineer Intervenes. Dr. John Edwards, University of Surrey; Mr. J. Steel, Nuffield Orthopaedic Centre; Mr. John MacLean, Eastman Dental Hospital.

A Self-maintaining Machine. Dr. Stephen Pelc, Medical Research Council; Miss Jennifer Tresise, School of Education, Reading University.

Telescoped Brains. Dr. Bernard Farrell, University of Oxford; Dr. George Mallen, Systems Ltd., Richmond.

Gods Themselves. Mrs. Micheline Vaughan, London School of Economics; Mr. W. Sheridan, School of Education, Reading University.

And those who, while not specially connected with any chapter, made it possible for me to get the books: Mr. Graham Geoghan and Mr. Graham Hatton, School of Education Library, Reading University.

D.F.J.

Contents

1

Current Views

In the past, man's dealings with death can be viewed in three phases. The first was the acceptance of it as a sacrosanct event, set up by an all-providing deity as a kind of gateway to paradise or damnation. This was man's view up until mediaeval times; it then passed to a second phase in which life was seen as a kind of legacy, a natural gift which could be spent or conserved according to whim.

The word 'natural' is significant here, because in the second phase man saw himself as possessing some control over the natural, but only the natural, span of life, provided all appropriate life-preserving techniques were used. Notable among these techniques (and in a sense we modern men are still half in this phase) were the medical and medico-social developments of antiseptic surgery, immunization, rational feeding and civic sanitation. If, in fact, the policy of this second phase were summed up in a few words, it might be said that man intended to 'give Nature a chance'.

When one reviews—however briefly—the course of these first two phases, one is not tempted to dramatization in any degree. For example, it would be an over-colourful thinker who described them as a battle with two antagonists, Man and Death, locked together. Yet the third phase, which is now beginning, does tempt just that kind of description, for it seems that grafting and transplanting surgery are already uniquely influencing man's earlier concept of death. For the first time, and here we need not concern ourselves with those nineteenth- and early twentieth-century attempts at glandular rejuvenation, man is not content to leave important body systems to deteriorate at what seems to be a pre-programmed rate. He is dissatisfied with the very marginal and inevitably overridden rewards, in terms of extended lifespans, which his second-phase efforts bring. So now for the first time he is attempting to break into the control box of life, and work the machinery for himself.

I am talking as if he were a single actor on a stage, but in fact, as the survey which follows shows, there is no such thing as a single attitude towards extended lifespans, except in the case of transplants, where some kind of unity of opinion is detectable. But transplants apart there is no such consensus, and thus it is misleading to talk about a battle in which collective man is on one side, and death is on the other. The situation is, in fact, much more complex.

However, consensus or not, attitudes to extended lifespans are important, not so much because their being positive or negative will necessarily make much difference to the prospects of man lengthening his life (the connection between technical innovation and public opinion is not as direct as that) but because they may give hints as to the way in which he will react to possible immortality, or virtual immortality in terms of personal and social readjustment.

At the moment man's prospects for longer life seem to depend upon the techniques of grafts and transplants, so obviously any study must include references to these. But with imagination one can also construct a scenario of future technical innovations against which a range of current attitudes can be tested by means of a questionnaire.

Transplants

The scenario runs thus. From now on, and by 'now' is meant this very year, the number of spare-part operations may be expected to increase, as will the frequency of success in terms of longer and longer survivals, despite the current fuss surrounding the most recent transplant deaths. National prestige, which seems to be waiting around for new outlets, preferably ones not tied to massive industrial power, may well latch on to the prospects offered by the transplant vogue, and deliver its own decisive shove to the whole process.

We may also expect that the struggle to find donors will push research more and more into sophisticated artificial-organ substitutes, notably hearts, arteries, kidneys and livers. Yet despite these successes certain frustrations and rethinkings may occur. Some cosmetic organ substitutions like massive skin grafts, for example, may not pass close cost/benefit scrutiny—people may find the treatment worse than the disease. Then again the ultimately palliative nature of organ renewal may not satisfy man's growing wish to prevent ageing rather than cure it temporarily. There may well also be a post-thermonuclear war emergency, in which a great proportion of the population finds itself sterile, and thus disposed to more radical ventures.

Halts

For these sorts of reasons attempts at halts (by which is meant the stopping of the overall process of bodily ageing) may be made. At the present time the actual proceedings for this halting are very uncertain. I think we can be fairly sure, however, that it will not be a once-for-all process. It is more likely to be similar to a regular 'servicing' except that each time the servicing occurs the deterioration that has taken place in the interval will be reversed. By this time it will be clear that the human body is the closest approach to a self-maintaining machine known, and that the gap between self-maintenance and decline can be narrowed or closed. Even limited narrowings of this gap will have substantial consequences in terms of enlarging the span of life, though whether halts will be permanent will be quite another matter. As regards popular pressure for halts, this may build up as soon as the inhibitions and cautions which stem from experience of normal lifetimes begin to die away. For by contrast transplant lifetimes will have had a feeling of normalcy about them.

However, halts, though successful in the biological and mechanical senses, will not be regarded as the final state, and the process will also come up against strong social and psychological pressures. Some of these, such as the problem of overpopulation, the food gap, and the tensions which may spring from 'selection-of-those-who-may-give-birth' situations, are obvious (or seem to be obvious) from our own point in time. But there may well be less obtrusive, and in the event more disturbing, pressures, some of which are hinted at in the answers which respondents gave to the survey.

Incorporations

Because of these pressures a third stage of extended lifespans may be anticipated which I have termed 'incorporations', meaning a merging of identities. In theoretical terms this process involves the physical transfer of ordered stores of information, complete with their identity components, from one brain to another. Now, if people show a willingness to be incorporated, thus defeating physical death by mental transfer, some of the more pressing social problems associated with halts, such as selection of those who can be allowed to give birth and narrow age-band populations, will disappear. At the same time, quite apart from the fact that incorporations may well throw up a fresh group of social difficulties, even such an advanced technique will not be the ultimate answer to the problem of mortality. There is a limited capacity in the human brain for taking in other identities, however reduced in scope. On the other hand, when we are dealing with an electronic system like the brain, our notions of space do have to undergo some stretching. Electrical dimensions are very much more elastic than our normal spatial sets, and the amount of data that can be packed within electrical space is enormous. In fact, true immortality will probably only be possible in a mechanical sense, and will involve the transfer of personal memories and identity to the memory stores of a computer.

In setting out this scenario I have skimmed over certain ideas and possibilities which I will examine at greater length in later sections. I ought to add, though, that the stages described – transplants, halts and incorporations – are not likely to be abrupt. On the contrary, a tapering in and out between them, or possibly some amalgamation of the techniques they demand, is to be expected.

THE QUESTIONNAIRE

With this scenario as a background, I constructed a questionnaire of twenty questions, angled at the emotional, social and physiological implications of the three main types of extended lifespan. In the question sequence the scenario's order of lifespan extension was very approximately retained, and the acceptability of each stage, whether transplants, halts or incorporations, was examined, the implications being then taken up in supplementaries. These were the twenty questions:

1. If you could have worn-out organs replaced, would you agree, even though the process could not be repeated indefinitely?

2. If you could be halted, in other words, have the process of bodily and mental ageing stopped, would you agree to undergo the process? And at what age would you choose to undergo it?

3. In a world of extended lifespans, parenthood might become a privilege. What might be the consequences of this?

4. Suppose a society in which all members were approximately the same age. Would this cause increased social friction, and in your opinion why?

5. Would you settle for an extended incorporate existence which narrowed down your personal identity to a single memory or skill?

6. Suppose you could be incorporated mentally with another person. What would be the important criteria for you? Incorporation within class, family, occupation, ethnic group or what?

7. How do you reassure yourself of your personal identity – by observing other people's reactions, by introspection, by recall, or by what means?

8. Have you ever felt a loss of identity in any sense?

9. Extended lifespans have been imagined as filled with boredom. Why do you think this opinion is held, and do you agree with it?

10. Some people might not want an extended lifespan. If you feel you might be in this group, please state your reasons.

11. These kind of speculations have been characterized as part of a modern phobia, similar to the sex phobia which we impute to the Victorians. Is this a glib dismissal in your yiew?

12. Suppose a mechanism were developed which increased the intensity of life at the cost of limiting its duration. Would you consider trying it?

13. We might look upon modern scientific research as being involved in the dualism, utter destruction or utter life. Which in your view is the most likely to win out in this conflict? Do you see it as a conflict?

14. Suppose you could live indefinitely, what 'priorities' would you set for recreation and achievement?

15. Space, Time and Death could be considered man's ultimate impediments. If the conquest of death involves the conquest of time, does the fact that man still has spatial bonds limit him, and if so, in what sort of ways?

16. Can you define in any coherent way your satisfaction, if you are satisfied, with the current fact of life's finite span?

17. Are there any special reliefs in bereavement? Have you felt emancipated in any way by bereavement? And would you regret a life in which there were no partings of this kind?

18. There may be basic satisfactions in living in a 'normal' age-spread population. Appropriate to your present age, what are these satisfactions?

19. Some people consider death to be a natural consequence, a terrifying prospect, a gateway to another life, a kind of deferred love affair, an exciting experience, or a humiliation. Which of these views do you hold, and why?

20. Knowing what you now know, does this sort of speculation frighten you, and if so, can you define your fright?

The fifteen respondents were asked to reply in writing, the broad outside limit for each answer being a hundred words, varying with the size of the respondent's handwriting. Some respondents regularly took all the space available for each question. Others replied with three- or four-word phrases or statements.

The first and most obvious comment to make about a group of articulate, well-informed, professional men and women, who would sit down to complete a twenty-item questionnaire, contribute individual totals of two thousand words, and submit themselves to questioning on a subject far removed from their own immediate concerns, is that they are not representative of the population as a whole.

Yet I am certain that any attempt to get an absolutely representative view on extended lifespans would be self-defeating. We shall see in the later analysis that there is considerable room for semantic confusion both in questions and answers – and short of writing an explanatory booklet on each question, this confusion will remain. At the same time, however, such woolly items do sometimes offer revealing oblique insights and speculations about mortality which might not be revealed in more straightforward questions. A multiple choice format might, therefore, produce a statistically impeccable but lifeless series of responses.

A second angle is that some of the ideas introduced in this survey are so speculative that they demand speculative respondents answering in open-ended situations. And it should also be pointed out that even if the results of this survey were held to be representative of the views of a liberal intelligentsia, nobody ought to go from this to claim that such attitudes and ideas must necessarily influence political decisions and choices, and therefore the prospects for extended lifespans.

We just do not know how the policy decisions are reached that determine which researches will take priorities, and quite apart from this there is plenty of evidence in the questionnaire that the respondents are keeping their options open. They tend, for example, to remark that they may feel differently about such and such a possibility if and when it ever comes about.

I know these caveats may seem to make the whole exercise somewhat academic. But this would be an over-depressive view. In the first place the psychological reactions of complex people to 'way-out' propositions are of interest because they may give an entirely new slant on traditional ideas and theories. Then again they may throw up ideas which can be tested out by further surveys or experiments. An instance of this is the response to the question of identity loss, which yielded a range of new and exploitable insights into the nature of identity.

ANALYSIS

As far as the analysis goes I felt I ought to begin with a test of the respondent's personal commitment to the questionnaire. The question I asked in an attempt to gauge this was, 'These kind of speculations have been characterized as part of a modern phobia, similar to the sex phobia which we impute to the Victorians. Is this a glib dismissal in your view?' (No. 11.)

This item was really a double test for it contained a very leaky analogy, which might have enabled the majority of the respondents to escape revealing their real attitudes. In fact, only a small proportion of the respondents dodged. Here is a dodger at work, however.

> 'I believe the equation is: Victorian view of sex = our view of death (both may be described as phobias). Any analogy leaks, and this one does too. I should not consider twentieth-century preoccupation with release from death (assuming it is a twentieth-century preoccupation) is in any way akin to middle- and upper-class Victorian *apparent* repression of sex.'

An equally small proportion openly considered the speculations were neurotic. But a heavy majority, possibly to be expected in view of the fact that the respondents had chosen to complete the questionnaire, thought that the speculations were rational, and gave this sort of reason.

> 'I think we must look ahead – we have got to do so in business, education, etc., and since change is so rapid it behoves us to speculate, so that we may help our children.'

I was also able to cast light upon another interesting facet of extended lifespans – the lack of discussion on the subject. I had always assumed that this verbal and oral silence must be due to some unacknowledged uneasiness. But at least, as far as these respondents went, this was not the case, for when I directly asked them if such speculation frightened them, and if so, whether they could define this fright (question No. 20), they overwhelmingly answered in the negative, and some of them chided me for being so naive as to expect them to be naive.

QUESTIONS RELATING TO TRANSPLANTS

As I have previously explained, the questions connected with methods of extending lifespans were tied closely with the sequence, transplants, halts and incorporations. The first specific question, therefore, was: 'If you could have worn-out organs replaced, would you agree, even though the process could not be repeated indefinitely?' (No. 1.)

Now, when I asked this question I expected an overwhelmingly negative response. The publicity of current heart-transplant attempts, the enormous but slightly diminishingly risk, the panoply of publicity-conscious surgeons, plus the hysterical atmosphere surrounding both donors and recipients, ought to have been sufficient to put off even the most hardened of would-be transplantees. But, of course, the question does not necessarily imply these things, and says nothing about this explicitly. Some transplants do not involve such horrifying risks, and kidney grafts have to be severely rationed.

In fact, the majority of the respondents had not been put off at all, and were willing to receive a transplant, provided certain conditions were met. For example, some wished to be sure about the prospects of organs other than those to be replaced by graft. The more humanitarian-seeming of them wanted to be reassured that a transplant for them would not mean a death for somebody else, and held firmly to the idea of artificial organs. They were also cautious. They tended to list specific transplant possibilities, keeping to eyes, kidneys, hearts and other vital organs, obviously judging the cosmetic and other possibilities of large-scale skin and hair transplants as not being worth the pain and discomfort involved.

Now the question about transplants was the only one specifically directed at this current bid for an extended lifespan. However, certain others, whose answers are to be analysed later, do touch upon the probable motivation for such an overwhelming acceptance of a novel technique. In the light of these the structure of the question itself, particularly the rider, 'the process could not be repeated indefinitely' must have been important. This, I am sure, must have given some respondents the reassuring feeling that in plumping for transplants they were not moving outside the limits of normalcy since they could visualize the life of a transplantee as not so outlandishly different in span from a conventional life. Such a transplant life might perhaps last a little longer, but not much longer, certainly not long enough to set off all those anxiety-provoking ideas that were released in response to later questions.

Secondly, transplants were probably seen as direct attacks upon physical decay. This is certainly a popular approach since the respondents seem to fear physical deterioration more than death. And then, probably as important although not as obvious is the cultural setting in which the question was framed. Within the respondent's experience there are of course no exact mechanical analogies to a self-maintaining machine (the possible effect of this in relation to halts will be discussed at greater length further on) but we do live in a 'tinkering culture'. In fact we have been steeped in the doctrine of repair from our earliest childhood, and only in our most recent years have we felt the beginnings of the 'buy it, use it, and scrap it' philosophy. Moreover, all these repairs going on all around us, to textiles, mechanisms and structures, have been carried out as if in response to strong moral, as well as economic precepts. Proverbs, for instance, have advised us that, 'a stitch in time saves nine'. The survey did not probe any deeper, but the subject of transplant attitudes is one which needs an extensive and meticulous research.

QUESTIONS RELATIVE TO HALTS

The next line of inquiry ran to attitudes towards halts, linking a direct question to this stage of the scenario. It asked, 'If you could be halted – in other words have the process of bodily and mental ageing stopped – would you agree to undergo the process? And at what age would you choose to undergo it?' (No. 2.)

Now if I had been asked to forecast the answer to these two questions, I would have been quite specific in predicting a heavy majority in favour of halting, and an equally heavy majority in favour of a halt age of about 20–25. But I would have been wrong on both counts.

In fact, there was an almost equal division between those willing, and those unwilling to undergo the halting process; and a range of reasons for these choices, which will emerge in later discussions. At the same time those willing to be halted did not choose their halt ages to my expected pattern. Few, at least, were prepared to exchange maturity for agility. The majority seemed, in fact, to prefer the marginal discomforts of early middle age (none of them actually opted for a halt in old age, however) to the mental stresses which they obviously associated with the emotional immaturity of youth. This meant, of course, that they were able to make a precise evaluation of personal satisfactions both physical and emotional, and select the age which gave them the best of both worlds. Here, for example, is a woman of late middle age expressing her willingness to be halted.

> 'This halting can only refer to the physical situation because living involves experience, from which we must learn. The age to choose, therefore, must be when all bodily functions are in

> perfect condition. One's senses must be alert, and one must be able to enjoy all forms of physical activity. The age of 25 would probably be satisfactory. If the social set-up were the same as I have lived through (which could not be), the age of complete independence from parents would have to be considered. To lead a satisfactory, self-chosen life, one must be free of control and obligation. As all people would be in the same situation, infirm parents would not exist. I would undergo the process.'

Note the interesting feature of her halt-age choice. It is true that, rather exceptionally, she chooses an early age, because as she says, she feels the need for absolutely untrammelled physical activity and expression. But despite this early choice, she too hankers after at least one of the emotional advantages of maturity – namely freedom from parental interference and ties.

This is the point too where the unrepresentative nature of the respondent group should be considered. Had they been labourers, for example, would they have been so willing to swop perfect agility for maturity? Might it not be the case that their intellectual roles have made them value marginal physical losses less than intellectual or emotional gains? Wielders of picks instead of pens might judge those physical declines more significant.

We must not forget the first part of the question, however, which caused a split between those who would and those who would not be halted. Here, in fact, we are at a very significant part of the questionnaire, because a pro or con answer can predict within reasonable limits the attitude the respondent will take to three other questions.

Before examining this split between halters and non-halters it might be as well to reconsider the 'tinkering culture' point made in relation to transplants. There is, of course, no true mechanical analogy to halts within the experience of the respondents. Self-maintaining machines as such do not exist, at least not in the sense in which each part of them consistently defies ageing or 'fatiguing'. Certain abstract mechanisms are conceivable, of course. By these I mean sophisticated organizations like modern industries which by dispersal or replacement can maintain themselves under economic stress or military attack. But it is unlikely that our respondents were thinking in these abstract terms. The lack of a true mechanical analogy to halts must be a factor, though indeterminate, in causing the halt and non-halt split, and it must operate by making the impracticable seem undesirable for some respondents.

Previously I mentioned three questions, the answers to which could be predicted on the basis of whether a respondent opted for or against a halt. These three 'splitting' questions have to do with the cohesion of a halt society, the problems of parenthood, and the nature of boredom in an extended lifespan.

In an attempt to assess the ways in which the respondents might view the cohesion of a halt society, I asked them to suppose one in which all members were approximately the same age, and to say whether this state of affairs would cause increased social friction, and why (No. 4).

Clearly most respondents took this question at its face value, assuming it to mean that physical age was the important variable involved, although it was also plain that a minority understood that even in a halt society people would be physically similar, but vary in the chronological length of their lives, and therefore possibly in their attitudes.

The majority clearly saw, and this in a sense is a tautology, that if there were no generations in a chronological sense, then there would be no conflict between them. But there was considerable ambivalence over such a conflict, some respondents viewing it as a stimulus or even a pleasure. Furthermore, some of those who foresaw peace emphasized that it might be bought at the cost of increased conflict within the single generation, since such a society would have few if any safety valves or outlets.

> 'I think that this would become unbearable, and would lead to increased social friction, since there would be no escape into, or opportunity to protest against, another age group. I am sure that age groups are complementary and give opportunity to observe coming age roles or look at them in retrospect through the young.'

> 'Decreased generation gap problem = less friction. But in a society such as this everyone would have the same objectives/aims, etc. = increased competition. Limited number of possibilities of achieving common aims = frustration = aggression = more friction. Probably the balance would fall on the side of increased friction. Also the problem of proving one's identity/individuality in a homogeneous (age-wise) society – depressing picture.'

On the whole those who would not consider being halted tended to emphasize the satisfactions of living in a normal-age-range population. What these satisfactions were, however, emerged in a later question, which did not divide halters from non-halters, and asked, 'There may be basic satisfactions in being in a normal-age-spaced population. Appropriate to your present age what are these satisfactions?' (No. 18.) From this direct assault four dominant themes of satisfaction emerged: variety, reflection, location and observation.

For variety we can distinguish two social forces which give pleasure. There is a horizontal force, the interaction of persons of similar ages, aims and interests; and there is the vertical, the cross-current of pressures exerted by the old and young on those in the middle. One gets a feeling that the respondents sense this dynamic lattice at work, and are satisfied by it. They find themselves at the centre of a complex social system, and specifically, this sense of location runs through a string of answers. They feel themselves anchored in the middle of a pattern of age groups, the boundaries of which are somewhat hazily defined by age, but which none the less are comfortingly existent. They enjoy their roles. They play their own with relish, and observe others playing those they have relinquished, an d the ones they will eventually assume. One respondent summed up this feeling very aptly.

> 'Young people can feel satisfied, older people wish they were young again. Middle people feel superior as old people are out of date, and young people haven't had their experience. Old people feel satisfied as they have seen/known more are wiser than the others because they desire death. At present have recently emerged from a dependence stratum – pleased to be (economically) self-supporting – looking forward to becoming a "supporter".'

It is as though in a Shakespearean sense they had the satisfaction of acting on the stage of life. But some were in the audience as well, and for them there was observation which was the delight in watching the development of children, presumably an opportunity to relive physical life vicariously, and possibly painlessly.

If we now go back to the second important question dividing halters and non-halters, we find it concerns that conventional response made to all speculations about the quality of an extended life, the assumption that it would be destroyed by boredom. Though it is banal the respondents' reaction to it was important, and so I angled the following question at it, 'Extended lifespans have been imagined as filled with boredom. Why do you think this opinion is held, and do you agree with it?' (No. 9.)

Now many of the respondents treated this as a challenge. It seemed to generate a kind of optimistic pride. Expected boredom, they maintained, was an artifact of unsatisfactory existences and the resultant inability to see extended or unlimited life except in such frustrating terms. The problems posed by senility, the restricting experience of suburban lifespans which multitudes could not escape, the 'one-job' lives, frequently in dull, unrewarding occupations, were all, they said, conditioning items which produced this kind of opinion. One of them summed it all up.

> 'A limited concept of a lifespan heavily conditioned by our experience of the past. It would appear to be largely self-fulfilling as we impose our own expectations upon each age barrier we reach. The economic need to "work" is one of the major conditionings (as opposed to "living") and education has played its part in the vicious circle of this conditioning.'

But if, manifestly and definitely, these people grasped the causes, they also held that they themselves were not bored. They had inner resources, a life plan, and further life was for most of them a continuous series of challenges which needed to be met, and even to be sought out. Manifestly and definitely, some of them declared they would not be bored with an extended lifespan, because if they were confronted with it, they would deploy the same inner resources to live it.

But there was a minority opinion that boredom was really only a screen (though not popularly understood as such) for a much deeper sickness. This malady, it declared, was not to be soothed by activity, because it arose from a doubt as to the purpose, rather than the lack or monotony, of doing. If this were the case (and these respondents tended to take a fatalistic view that there was no answer to this malady except death) then no amount of activity could stave off eventual boredom. A more sophisticated point made by some held that boredom is built into our life mechanisms, and that death in a sense is the natural answer to it.

The last of the dividing questions concerned a need basic to the human situation, that of parenthood. Any halt phase not accompanied by a quite extraordinary breakthrough in food production would inevitably involve some kind of birth control, if not direct permission to conceive. So I put the question, 'In a world of extended lifespans, parenthood might become a privilege. What might be the consequences of this?' (No. 3.)

It was probably the word 'privilege', and also perhaps because the subjects were too much children of their time to have responded differently, that caused this question to open up a series of 'brave-new-world' reactions. Two themes were closely intertwined: eugenics and state interference with the right of conception and procreation. Some of the respondents were very clear about the administrative mechanism of this interference, seeing the state compelled to discriminate in a most arbitrary and brutal fashion between would-be parents. They also went off at a tangent, visualizing an elaborate and obsessive drive to produce a superman, a venture which might or might not raise the intellectual level of the species, but would in their view increase the quota of human misery and frustration.

A second group, however, did not respond in quite such an emotional way to the word 'consequences', in the question. For them there obviously were going to be consequences, but they did not necessarily see them as malignant. In fact, though they mostly envisaged the same consequences, they were able to write about them in a more neutral way, as if less deeply affected by them, or able to come to terms with them. On the other hand, this neutral group was not provoked into throwing up any strikingly optimistic or benign speculations. For example, it did not suggest the possibility of 'parenthood by ballot', or conceive a society which could differentiate accurately between greater and lesser parental needs, or one which could arrange parenthood substitution.

On these three questions then, a kind of discriminating profile of the halt versus the non-halt respondent could be built. In general terms the halt individual seems to be less convinced that the maintenance of society's existing age-range pattern is a necessary ingredient for human happiness. He does not seem to be anxious about the prospects of fresh instinctual restraints for different social circumstances, possibly because he has small gratification from those particular instincts, and also perhaps because he believes that freshly created instinctual gratifications, possible in a new society, would appeal to him more. He tends not to think of extended lifespans as boring, being confident in his own internal resources, and having personally proved to himself within his own limited lifetime that he can defeat such boredom.

The non-halt individual, on the other hand, sees little profit in this supposed piece of human re-engineering with its considerable social consequences. In fact he sees a loss. More than the halt individual, he tends to take a gloomy view of the prospects of a halt society, being much concerned with the overriding consequences of strife within the single generation, while at the same time conceding that there might be an easing of intergenerational tensions. And he is concerned about boredom in an extended lifespan.

It needs to be emphasized that these variations in attitude do not mean a clear-cut line-up for the three significant questions. Because an individual respondent is a non-halter, it does not follow that he or she will show three consistent apprehensions for the three questions or vice versa. All the same a divisive tendency is particularly marked in these three, which prompts a query as to whether the difference is anchored to basic differences in attitude, or accidental in the sense in which the initial choice (halt or non-halt) is according to whim, and the subsequent split comes about because this initial choice has to be rationalized.

The latter possibility is unlikely, I feel. A rationalization of such a kind would be bound to extend further into the questionnaire than it does. There are in fact a half-dozen very loaded questions still to be analysed, which could show the dichotomy. But they do not do so.

For instance, this dichotomy does not emerge in any attempt to discover what the respondents would *do* with their extended lifespans. To delve into this problem the group was asked, 'Suppose you could live indefinitely, what "priorities" would you set for recreation and achievement?' (No. 14.)

Now, despite the fact that this question was academic to those who had declared themselves against an extended lifespan, almost all respondents answered it fully and imaginatively, generally under one or more of three major headings: perfection, experience, and service.

Under perfection we can group all kinds of speculations about the possibilities of developing expertise in mental, manipulative, creative or social fields. And it was in this category that the respondents showed for the first time their potential for thinking with a full command of their imaginations. A whole range of such skills was suggested, some as yet untried, and others showing unacceptably low levels of achievement.

> 'Studying for other professions, particularly medicine and psychiatry. Mastering other languages. Exploring remote lands,

understanding foreign cultures. Skiing, skating, climbing. Being as efficient with an aeroplane as with a car. Making things from metal, wood and clay. Making my own clothes. Gardening. Repeating ideal moments with friends new or old: a moonlight beach barbecue after swimming in a tropical sea; sun glitter sparkling on the sea, broken by green mountainous islands, and eating exotic food; a service in a Lutheran church in Sweden, candle lit, with strong arches disappearing into huge blackness; climbing the Chancellor Ridge in mist; roasting chestnuts while the wind and rain howl outside; sensing male strength.'

But of course, most of the respondents have been steeped in the aptitude-level doctrine which set limits of achievement for skills. For them to go beyond this framework in their speculations means either that they no longer accept the doctrine, or that they are confident that the effects of indefinitely extended practice will invalidate it, or that they believe in the efficacy of as yet unexplored teaching methods.

A theologian would identify this quest for perfection as a kind of modern, self-inflicted purgatory – a purging not so much of sins, but of inadequacies. Purgatory was traditionally conceived of as a phase of preparation for a fuller and more perfect after life – the sinner or imperfect one being prepared to measure up to cosmological or eternal yardsticks. Our respondents are still thinking, of course, in terms of yardsticks. But in a way they are preparing themselves not so much to meet God as to meet themselves. I am not, incidentally, suggesting here that they are in the process of deifying themselves in an absolute sense. Indeed the question does not prompt this. Extended lifespans are still lifespans, they are not absolute immortality.

But if we take another, 'Space, time and death could be considered man's ultimate impediments. If the conquest of death involves the conquest of time, does the fact that man still has spatial bounds limit him, and if so, in what sort of ways?' (No. 15) and analyse the answers to this, then we find that only a small minority of respondents consider space as a definite limitation of man. And they are heavily outnumbered by those who

a. see space as an entirely notional and unimportant impediment; or
b. see it as a way in which man is defined, but do not admit or deny it as an impediment; or

c. agree that if space is dependent on the time/distance ratio, and one side of the ratio no longer holds, then space hangs on nothing.

Combine these two responses, Nos. 14 and 15, and they seem to show that although some respondents are not willing to go the whole way, and consider themselves as the equal of God, they are prepared to picture themselves as having a subordinate godlike status. And in some theologies there are models for this. The Greeks had demigods and the Christians have their angels.

I next tried to discover whether the respondents rebelled against death, or yielded to it willingly, by asking them, 'Can you define in any coherent way your satisfaction, if you are satisfied, with the current fact of life's finite span?' (No. 16.)

The key word in this question turned out to be 'satisfied'. But it caused evasions, because in this context it is really meaningless. Dissatisfaction is possible only in circumstances when a more satisfactory alternative is available, and the only consequence of asking respondents whether they were satisfied with the inevitable was to draw out from most of them strategies or rationales concerned with their adjustment to, or acceptance of death. With one exception, the respondents did not define their satisfaction in any way coherent or otherwise – they wrote about their acceptance, and they revealed the essential contingency of that acceptance.

In other words they constantly reiterated their acceptance of the finite span of life, because it was the same for everybody, and the normal order of things. They used this universality as a kind of bandage, to cover an incessantly tender spot, and by and large it did its prophylactic job, that is, it prevented their speculating too hard and too long on the inevitability of death. But, of course, it is a bandage not an ideology. It means that they will continue to accept, as long as the traditional order of living is undisturbed, and as long as everyone comes under the same regime. But if exceptions should ever occur, this acceptance may be expected to transform itself into rejection, because our respondents are not *satisfied* with mortality as such, they are only satisfied with their adjustment to it.

However, if they seemed only superficially adjusted to the idea of their own deaths, they were more positive about the 'value' of other people's. When they were asked, 'Are there any special reliefs in bereavement? Have you felt emancipated in any way by bereavement? And would you reject a life in which there were no partings of this kind?' (No. 17) the positive response was very dominant.

With some, the motivation was directly humanitarian.

> 'There is I suppose some purifying force in grief. There is a special relief in bereavement when the subject is released from suffering either physical or mental.'

And in others, the pleasure principle was much to the fore.

> 'Yes – what, lose the self-satisfaction of grief? You must be joking. One of the few occasions in the twentieth century where the individual is socially permitted total self-indulgence.'

And in others, bereavement seemed to be valued for its part in ensuring social variety.

> 'I feel certain there are reliefs related possibly to seeing the *conclusion* of a life which has brought more happiness than grief to other men. Conclusion of a stage or chapter which must necessarily end before another can begin. Life is a continuous cycle of endings and beginnings and partings, and to regret them or to still them is to wish a form of stagnation or crystallization.'

My penultimate question in the halt field was, 'Some people might not want an extended lifespan. If you feel you might be in this group please state your reasons' (No. 10). In fact this is a good example of the way in which intentions can be misunderstood, if essential contexts are omitted. The attempt here was to test out the possibilities of 'life martyrdom', in other words, to anticipate the existence of men and women who, given a choice of taking an extended lifespan or dying in a natural way, would choose to die. Whether the 'life martyr' will appear or not, the attempt failed because the respondents took the question as a restatement of the earlier 'would you be halted' item, and echoed or referred to their earlier answer.

But not everyone. In some there was a significant change. For whereas at the earlier point there had been a majority (though very slight) for halts, the situation was now reversed. This would indicate that the questionnaire with ten items delving into the implications of extended lifespans had its own effect on attitudes. To be more specific, it may have pushed over some respondents from the camp of the uncommitted to the camp of the negatives.

So that although in one respect the question is a failure, it shows nevertheless that even in this novel field, attitudes can be shifted in the course of a questionnaire by a close analysis of the facts. But it also shows that some people are not so flexible, and are in a sense committed by existing attitudes to an acceptance of extended lifespans.

Finally as a contribution to no special category of extended lifespans I decided to test out the 'crowded hour' hypothesis. We all know the poetic assertion that 'one crowded hour of glorious life is worth an age without a name'. Poets and others have made this claim so confidently, and some of the respondents were so adamant that chronological time was not to be equated with living in the fullest sense, that I wondered how far they were prepared to take this denial. In particular I wanted to know if the most vociferous 'time not living' respondents were, in fact, time bound. So I put the question, 'Suppose a mechanism were developed that increased the intensity of life at the cost of limiting its duration, would you consider trying it?' (No. 12.)

With the single exception of a consistent hair splitter, who maintained his consistency by challenging the word 'intensity' and then declaring the question meaningless, all respondents answered in the negative. Some were strident in declaring that life was too intense as it was; others were more analytical, discussing the problems of heightened sensation, questioning the logical possibility of a universal increase in intensity of experience, or the curious consequences of some people leading more intense lives than others. But threading through all the negative answers, short and long, I had a sense of touching upon something very basic in the human psyche. This must be a very deep feeling of chronological entitlement – a feeling which is in itself a satisfaction, that one is allowed a certain amount of time to live within. Poets are supposed to be greater realists than scientists, but it would seem that they are not so much realists as extremists. The respondents, it is true, do not by and large live nameless ages. But even if they were living such lives, they seem unwilling to trade the nameless age for the crowded hour. A crowded hour is conceptualized as an hour, regardless of how crowded it is, and even the most vociferous of the 'time not living' respondents respect time as a real entity.

QUESTIONS RELATING TO INCORPORATIONS

We now come to the responses to the last phase of the scenario, incorporations. The first, and probably key question in this was,

'Would you settle for an extended, incorporate existence which narrowed down your personal identity to a single memory or skill?' (No. 5.)

Now this was a very basic probe, which should have drawn out the respondents' view of their own 'selfness', the bond that they had made with the central core of their beings. Questions unasked, but allied to it at greater or lesser distance, were whether identity was synonymous with memory, and if so whether a single memory, could carry the weight of a self. Central was the problem of visualizing a state of incomplete identity, and I expected that difficulties in thinking about this would be touched on in any lengthy responses that were given.

In fact, few responses were lengthy, and with a single exception they were tightly explicit, and adamant that they would have none of this incorporate existence. But in the answers that were not simple negatives, some sharp insights into the nature of 'selfness' were offered.

> 'I am unable to visualize myself without my complete hotch-potch of pecularities, memories and abilities, good and bad. To become part of some multiple-minded being would not be me. I need to be in control. Unsatisfactory traits need improving; I must choose which, and how. A reason for living is to strive to change certain parts of my entity until I can approve of them. The suggestion of narrowing my identity is intolerable. I must be all or nothing.'

> 'No – because I should no longer be a person in the fullest sense, I would only be a machine.'

Existence, without the complete entity they had learned to call themselves was plainly out of the question. I seemed to have uncovered a hitherto unarticulated equation, an iron equation that did not admit of any tampering, which held that the reason for existence was to savour identity and its elaborations, and further required that identity together with its elaborations must be complete.

I tried to come closer to this concept of identity in a second question, 'Have you ever felt a loss of identity in any sense?' (No. 8.) This is, of course, another semantically dubious item, so before we see how the respondents answered it, it might be as well to review its psychological implications. If we equate loss of identity with the feelings of not being oneself, then psychiatry knows this as a part of various mental illnesses. Such feelings occur in anxiety states, depressions, and in amnesias involving loss of memory for name or other personal details. At a more critical level, the onset of schizophrenia is often accompanied by such feelings, which in these cases may precede delusions and general fragmentation of the personality.

This is a loss of identity within emotional illness, but feelings of depersonalization and derealization can and, if the respondents' records are anything to go by, do occur frequently in the near-normal state. In these cases they take the form of ruminations about reality, or fleeting feelings of not being oneself.

It was clear that a substantial group of respondents had experienced these sensations, usually in childhood or adolescence, that they had disliked them, and that they did not want to repeat them. Their answers seem to show that identity loss, even though not experienced in a neurotic or psychotic setting, is anxiety-provoking on its own account.

Here are some typical responses to the loss item.

> 'Yes – often in early adolescence – it took the form of an acute introspection. For brief finite periods I wondered who I was – then "unselfconsciousness" would return.'

> 'Yes – momentarily and rather frighteningly I have felt my identity slipping away from me (this sometimes happens when I dwell on my name for some time).'

Another point which came up relates closely to the theory that some people's personal identity seems to hinge upon group affiliation. A respondent stated why he had never lost his identity.

> 'Not at all, because I've always been part of *small* institutions, even during my service in R.A.F.'

In this case too great a multiplication of relationships seems to be the threat, so the respondent has taken pains to keep them as limited as possible. This might be another possible clue to the general anxiety expressed over incorporations – a multiplicity of internal relationships in an incorporated state being too much for the average identity to contemplate.

It is also clear that the respondents all believe in personal free will. The philosophy came peeping out of a range of responses.

Although the survey does not deal with this aspect of cognition, external evidence would suggest that when it comes to other minds, respondents see these as the reverse of free, and very much in the grip of external causations. This is little more than speculation, but perhaps the respondents do not welcome incorporation, because they fear it would destroy their very carefully nourished belief in 'free will'. Machines or robots are not free. And it is the machine or robot they say they might become, if they allowed themselves to be incorporated.

For clarity I feel I ought to summarize these anxieties in tabulated form.

a. They see no reason to go on living, if they cannot be themselves.
b. They are afraid of their old experiences of identity loss.
c. They dislike multiple relationships, a threat they avoid in a one-body existence.
d. They value their own control, however illusory, and fear that they will find it illusory if they ever come to be incorporated.

And yet despite the fact that they cling to themselves as a policy, they seem to be vague on methods to test their identity. When they were asked, 'How do you reassure yourself of your personal identity – by observing other people's reactions, by introspection, by recall, or by what means?' (No. 7) – there was, of course, a sub-group of Cartesians who hitched themselves solidly to the fact of conscious thought. But the majority outside that circle held none of the identity tests as sovereign, and mostly wrote in terms of a flux of all three, and more besides.

> 'By all of the above in a way which relates them. They are systematically organized, it appears, and the external stimulation of one will set some or all of the others in motion. I do grade people and their reactions in degrees of importance. Some people's reactions are more important, but their reactions when they are in some emotional states (e.g. anger) or in some physical states (e.g. pain) I consider irrelevant.'

Finally, if they are pressed to ponder the actuality of incorporation they can be led into an interesting paradox. The last identity question asked, 'If you could be incorporated mentally into another person, what would be the important criteria for you?

Incorporation within class, family, occupation, ethnic group, or what?' (No. 6.)

From this came a range of choices. Some were not within the criteria suggested. But a large majority plumped for ethnic grouping, which is not surprising in one sense, since it is known that large numbers of people relate intimately to their culture, and see in cultural compatibility a method of preserving their own identity.

And yet one would have expected that all these respondents, including the minority without the conventional liberal restraints, would have been sufficiently conditioned by recent integration propaganda to have avoided revealing racialist-type choices. How is it then that a significant number of them make this ethnocentric selection? Revealingly, at another point, a respondent identified the sexual act as a sort of incorporation. One wonders if, at a deeper mental level, incorporation is in fact identified as a kind of sexual intercourse, which kicks off those species-selection mechanisms that racial conflict tends to rouse. Under normal interrogation our respondents might make liberally affirmative answers to the question, 'Would you let your daughter marry a coloured man?' When it comes to their own incorporations, they face the same unconscious pressures but without the liberal conditioning to guide them to make the liberal reply.

Yet another feature of response to this item is its essential cautiousness. That caution is frequently a respondent characteristic must be obvious from previous responses. But in terms of incorporative criteria they are here seeking absolute compatibility before anything else. They do not look for excitement, creativity or contrast. They do not suggest incorporations with members of the opposite sex, with artists, engineers, intellectuals, or men of action. It is as though the product of forcing them to consider this phase has tripped off their most conservative instincts, and induced them to give only the most grudging of choices.

In the final summing up: this survey deals with chances. If we observe man's activities, it would seem that our death-dealing and our life-preserving efforts may both spring from the same source, namely *the struggle to survive on our own terms.* Paradox piles on paradox here. Immortality could come about as an accidental spin-off from, say, a nerve gas, found to have limitless tissue-preservative properties. On the other hand we might discover in our search for immortality a wonder drug which eliminated bone and cartilage fatigue, but which when atomized became a devastating new weapon in bacteriological warfare. This is the dualism of man's technological destiny and in a question I put the possibilities to the respondents as sharply as possible.

The question asked, 'We might look upon modern scientific research as being involved in one dualism, utter destruction or utter life. Which in your view is more likely to win out in this conflict? Do you see it as a conflict?' (No. 13.)

Once more there was the usual quota of semantic dodging. There were those who objected to my seeming to load the onus for choice upon the scientist (which I had not). There were those who professed ignorance of 'utter destruction', and were even more foggy about 'utter life'. There were those who claimed that since life was founded upon destruction, the question was meaningless. But the majority was optimistic. They hardly knew what 'utter life' meant, but they seemed to have a kind of confidence that it would come out on top in the end (whatever the end might be, and however far off).

2

Not All Their Own

This section is concerned with transplants and the ways in which they may affect the mortality of man. It represents the second part of man's four-phase assault on death. We live in effect at the beginning of the transplant age, and the beginnings of anything are seldom if ever based upon plans or strategies. Indeed, the beginnings of innovations usually involve crisis situations (as in heart surgery), palliatives or short-term solutions. And yet we can see several ways in which transplants may develop from the stage of being crisis or stop-gap measures to become part of a long-term policy of organ renewal.

In this policy, as in many others, two factors must be balanced. The first is long-term gain, and the second immediate discomfort. In therapeutic terms, is the operation worth the pain and inconvenience that beings suffer? In transplants, however, neither is a constant. They are variable because, on the one hand, engineering progress is making artificial implanted organs more efficient every day, while at the same time, but on a slower scale, surgery is becoming more refined, and less traumatic.

It is an interesting paradox that in such a mechanical age, the first organ transplants (apart from bone shafts) should have been natural and not artificial. The first actual grafting done in surgery was autograft skin (transferring skin from one site to another on the same body), which was a mediaeval technique. Homograft transplants (donor to recipient) began with kidneys in the twentieth century. The first organ to catch the headlines was the human heart, and it was the human heart that first showed up the two great problems of grafts, rejection and preservation.

In fact, the essential problem in all transplants whether artificial or natural is how to suppress the rejection phenomena that almost inevitably appear within a few days, weeks or months of a successful surgical introduction of a foreign organ. The best-tried and most successful drugs so far used to combat rejection have been Predisnolone and Imuran. But both these agents have curious and in some cases dangerous side effects. For example, Asiatics are hypersensitive to both, and in some cases will develop gastric ulcers when given amounts that would cause no harm to Europeans. There may also be tie-ups between these immunosuppressive drugs and lowered resistance to the development of infections. It is of course realized that the lymphocytes (lymph cells) play a major part in marshalling the rejection forces, and the immunosuppressive drugs do, in fact, immobilize these, and keep them from attacking the graft. Unfortunately they weaken every other resistance point as well, whether concerned with the graft or not.

If, however, a substance is introduced into the lymph stream that will destroy the lymphocytes alone, and not spread all over the body, then the doses of immunosuppressive drugs can be kept to a minimum. Japanese physiologists have perfected a method of injecting radioactive gold into the lymph system, which acts in just such a way. It kills lymphocytes, keeps itself to itself, and does not irradiate the tissues dangerously. If subsequent experience supports the success of earlier trials it should be a valuable corrective to immunosuppressive therapy.

The second big problem in all transplants involving natural organs, whether taken from living donors or corpses, is preservation. Donors may die far away from recipients; there may be pre-operative delays caused by the health of both donors and recipients; in fact there are a myriad possible complications that can delay the actual grafting. Gradually, however, the various factors that combine to keep a graft alive in the period between removal from donor and transfer to recipient have been identified.

These factors seem to be temperature, pressure and the nutrition of the graft while it is in disembodied isolation, factors that can only be adequately satisfied in a special machine. And as all these factors must be satisfied in combination, it is of little use leaving any out.

The importance of these requirements became very clear during the first heart transplants. We now know heart transplantation to be a very risky surgical venture, at least when measured against the actual numbers of transplant heart survivals.

Of course we do not know, and have no means at present of knowing, how far the small number of survival successes and the large number of failures might compare with the recovery/death rate of patients selected for grafts, had they not received them. In fact, there is no doubt that to be selected for heart-transplant surgery is almost synonymous with a surgical decision to try anything since death seems otherwise inevitable.

At the same time there is an interesting discrepancy between the success of heart grafts in dogs, and its relative failure in humans. In a relatively high proportion of dog heart transplantations the dogs seem to have survived, and have suffered neither rejection crises nor serious deterioration in their capacity for living.

With hearts particularly we seem to be faced, as indeed we are to some extent in the cases of liver and lung grafts, with an organ of primary significance, one whose efficiency is vital in the success of grafts of every kind. It is, therefore, not likely to be easy to graft an organ of this status.

We are also faced, as we are with brain grafts, with deep difficulties in the preparation of the graft itself, in that the donor cannot function without it, this necessity interfering with the viability of the organ to be transferred. And finally there is the problem of the condition of the organ itself, which may often only be obtained after a devastating accident which the victim does not survive, and which must damage all parts of him, in subtle if not obvious ways.

Generally the same remarks apply to attempts which have been made to transplant lungs. During the past fifteen years there has been a considerable amount of work done on lung transplantation, and it is probably true to say that at least as far as surgical techniques go, the ways in which lungs can be grafted are known as well as they need to be known for success in this aspect of the operation. Unfortunately surgical technique, though important, is only one factor in lung transplants.

Of greater significance is the physiological effects of transplantation, in other words all the phenomena of rejection, which seem to be particularly violent in the case of lungs. It is interesting to note that in many cases where organs other than lungs have been grafted, lungs have been the first sites to show signs of rejection by suddenly becoming inflamed. A syndrome known as 'transplant lung' has been named as a frequent consequence of grafting operations.

With this sensitivity to other grafts as an indicator, it is hardly surprising that lungs should be particularly difficult to transplant themselves. Another measure of this sensitivity is the quite extraordinary difference in success rate between autografts and homografts. Autografts, lung transplants exchanging the subject's own lungs, have been tried, principally on animals, but also on man, and the results have been very encouraging. A high percentage of autografted animals survived, and approximately 75 per cent of the human patients.

But it is an entirely different picture with homografts. In terms of animal subjects, it is very difficult to stretch survival beyond a year, and in humans the picture is a good deal grimmer. Of the dozen or so men who have had transplants, not one has survived longer than four weeks, although in several cases the rejection of the graft did not kill the patients because they survived on one lung.

It is also fairly clear that because of the risks of the operation, surgeons can expect very few lungs from live donors, which means that the future of the operation depends on grafts from corpses, and this introduces several very difficult though familiar obstacles. The lungs of cadavers are particularly likely to have been damaged by the process which led to the donor's death. It is also very difficult to clean out a cadaver lung in a comprehensive way that will ensure its not carrying debris which will set up complications in its new site.

It may well be of course that sophisticated tissue matching, improved methods of damping down rejection reactions, and ways of enhancing tolerance will eventually make both natural lung and heart transplantation better prospects than they are at present. It is certainly very true that heart or lung defects are a very significant cause of death whether they manifest themselves in obvious and fatal conditions like cancers or clots, or in the more subtle circulatory changes that put insupportable pressures on other organs. But this must inevitably place great demands on the somewhat dubious supply of natural grafts. In this situation, can we expect an artificial heart/lung machine, or is this technically impossible?

What kind of machine would it be? We already have large, heavy heart/lung machines which are used as by-pass oxygenators in operations. Fundamentally, of course, an implant could consist of two miniature pumps driven by two motors, one pump to handle the lung, and the other to handle the heart function. But the two motors would need to be of a most sophisticated design. They would need to be coupled together with a complex gear/

clutch linkage which would allow one to assist the other in time of breakdown; and in addition to this each individual motor would need to be segmentally built, in other words its connective and brush systems would be sectionalized in order to make it more reliable. Both would be so arranged (as in Fig. 1) that each could be disconnected so that, while possibly reducing the blood or air pumping to an uncomfortable level, it would not be dangerous to the patient, and both would allow temporary drives to be coupled up while either was off shaft for repair. Their lubrication would be of an advanced boundary type, not dependent upon external supplies of lubricant, but built into the bearing systems themselves. They would have miniaturized monitoring devices at all wear and fracture points, which would be set to transmit warnings of possible fractures whenever they sensed changes in the part to which they were attached.

As to the moving parts themselves, or other parts that might come under stress, these would be fabricated with immense care. All the vast modern developments in whisker construction, anti-crack, composite materials, plus the most minute examination of surfaces and interiors by X-ray crystallography techniques, would be used in their construction. And they would need to be near noiseless, and very carefully balanced in regard to their torque or gyroscopic effects. Such problems might be eased by the use of two motors and two pumps, an arrangement which could be designed to balance out some or all of these particularly disturbing phenomena. The linkage of motors and pumps could resemble the diagram in Fig. 1, with each unit inter-

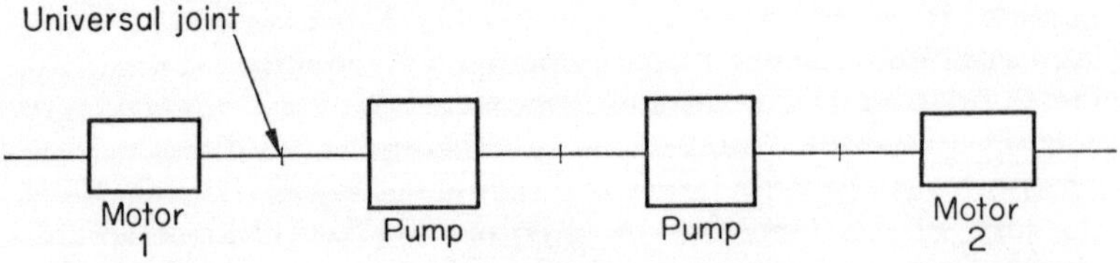

Fig. 1

coupled on a common shaft with universal joints to give a more convenient positioning. Both Motor I and Motor II would be spliced on to the common shaft, so that either could be withdrawn for servicing or replacement if necessary.

Two problems which could arise from an array of this kind might be *a*. the production of trapped gases from the brush systems of the motors, and *b*. the extra weight and power losses arising from the necessity to convert rotational motion to reciprocation (in the case of pulse-type blood pumps).

These two problems at least could be eliminated by using a motor of the solenoid kind. This is essentially a piston electric motor utilizing the expulsion effect in an energized coil of a bar of metal within it. The diagram in Fig. 2 shows such a motor.

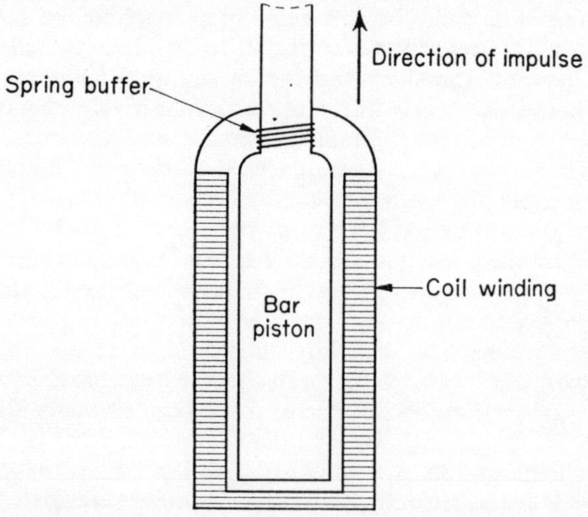

Fig. 2

A vertically mounted coil, prewound, at right-angles to the mounting, surrounds a cylinder in which runs a piston. Intermittent pulses of current are fed to the coil which cause the piston to jump upwards against the recoil of a spring. The reciprocating motion is transmitted directly to a pulse-type blood pump.

This system eliminates at a stroke a whole train of complicated gearings, joints and contacts, and at the same time reduces wear since the piston is only in frictional contact intermittently at the floor and spring end of the cylinder.

One of the big problems would be fixing. An implant heart-lung machine, although manufactured of materials such as carbon fibre or fibre glass, would weigh an appreciable amount. It might also vibrate to a limited degree, and perhaps give off some heat as a by-product of its function. Yet it would be difficult to anchor it to any of the more obvious structures of the body, such as the rib cage. A vibrating weight pinned to a rib might seem to be an excellent method of arranging matters, but bones respond in curious and dramatic ways to having weights fixed to them. Build-ups of bone take place around pins or ties, due possibly to the electrical effects of metal in contact with bone. And thus what would seem to be an excellent fixture might well turn out to create a very serious mis-shaping of the bone anchor itself.

If the diaphragm (that muscular sheet at the base of the lungs) were used as a floor for the heart-lung machine – a possibility only – a very carefully custom-designed packing would have to be put between the sides and top of the device and the thorax wall, allowing a certain amount of play, but also ensuring that the machine did not vibrate too much and thus fracture its connecting pipes. This packing could well be in the form of a sponge plastic (it could not be anything inflatable, for fear of puncture) which would have to be modelled to fit the individual patient's thoracic cavity. It might have to be sectionalized also, to allow for the passage of pipes and leads, which would also give it the necessary flexibility to permit normal trunk movements.

It hardly needs to be added that such a plastic presents a universe of design problems in itself. It would have to be at one and the same time soft, strong, absolutely air-tight and easily mouldable, to say nothing of being non-inflammable. It might need to be prepared at some speed, and yet keep these characteristics. Finally it would have to be relatively cheap.

Power supply for the inbuilt heart-lung machine is also important. The human heart takes approximately four watts of power for its normal beating programme, and a watt or so more when it is under heavy load. The lungs' requirements are approximately the same, but again demand rises when load increases. While we are very unlikely to be able to match the heart's efficiency as a pump by mechanical means, and will therefore have to face up to a high power requirement for the mechanical replacement, it is possible that cutting down on some cardiac luxuries may give a wattage saving. A source inside the body of some 10–12 watt power will therefore be required.

As to cardiac luxuries it is worth observing that man has one great advantage as far as design goes. Entering the design field, millions of years late as it were, he does not have to build 'animal contingency' into his designs in the same way as Nature has had to do. It is not necessary to equip a business man's heart with the complex feeds and shunts that will enable him to beat a lion to the barrier if one appears on the 8.15, because the chances of such a happening are infinitely remote. Man as a designer is dealing with a rational animal (or at least his responsibilities as a designer may be assumed to be at an end when man becomes irrational). He can therefore dispense with much of the evolutionary design baggage that nature has not had time to off-load.

Where can the heart-lung designer derive his power supplies? There are three possible alternatives. He can use a thermocouple, that is he can directly translate bodily heat into electricity; he can tap the bones for their considerable voltage; or he can use the chemical contents of the body to form a gigantic battery. None of these will be easy supplies to arrange, however. The introduction of the necessary components to build the batteries may cause adverse reactions with the body. Bones may object to being tapped, thermocouples may be rejected. And all three sources of power may be needed to boost output, which may mean that they will react together adversely.

There is, in fact, one other way of providing power without loading the body with external attachments, and this is to insert short-duration power packs. These are already developed for various other commercial uses, and usually involve a high-voltage input for a short period, which the battery expends at a low-voltage output. All the commercial designs involve direct coupling, which might be possible if external lead connections could be maintained on the surface of the body. But it may become practicable to energize the battery indirectly, that is by placing the subject in a field of electrical energy which can be picked up within his body. Sleeping within this field, with the subject's bed as the high-energy field, might be practicable, and thereby a nightly recharge could be taken without inconvenience.

The specification for the heart pump is also a very demanding one. In essence what is required is a two-phase pump, one phase of moderate capacity to handle the current of blood through the lungs (or the artificial lungs) and the other of greater power to drive the oxygenated blood round the rest of the body. A second important consideration is the actual continuity of the flow, which in normal circumstances is of pulse pattern, and may have to be designed for in that way because many other body systems are used to it. And a third important point is the relationship between the two phases, which must not be allowed to get out of balance, as it were. In other words, blood supply needs must equal, at all times, oxygen provision.

Turbo-pumps which use storage vessels to give the correct intermittency to their thrust, or pulse pumps which depend on piston or squeeze movements, are still in the process of development for the heart function. Unfortunately they consume much power, which at this moment of primitive technology would probably mean that they would have to rely upon an external source like a portable battery pack or compressed-air cylinder. A second problem is that they do a lot of damage to the blood itself.

Blood is a complicated and delicate substance, and it is very averse indeed to being bundled through rotors at high speeds, or squeezed unendurably in high-pressure cylinders. Such treatment (it suffers some damage in fact from the pumping action of the natural heart) alters its density, and ruptures the cases of its red cells. It is for this reason that an artificial heart pump has been designed which does not actually work with blood itself, but indirectly through a transmitted impulse. Much of the soft chamber system of the heart is retained, but inside is contemplated a turbo-pump pulsator which transmits its pulse to the blood by expanding and contracting an envelope filled with liquid, thus forcing the blood in and out of the usual outlets. Fig. 3 shows this idea in very simple form.

Although the diagram does not cover all aspects this is a very sophisticated device indeed, because in one unit it answers the needs of the system in terms of

a. the dependency of one phase on another (because among other things the pulsator can organize its output to balance up body demand with oxygen supply);
b. the fact of pulse itself, because it creates an artificial pulse;
c. the elimination of any contact between the delicate blood and tough inorganic parts, except for that portion of the envelope which touches the bloodstream.

Unfortunately it is not simply the problem of blood damage from artificial parts that exercises the engineer. Blood has enormous clotting capacity, a capacity which is demonstrated not only in the healing of wounds but also when blood comes into contact with foreign materials. Valves, ducts, turbine-blades, shafts and filters may all trigger off this clotting, a problem which may make heart/lung implant maintenance a nightmare. Its solution is indeed very difficult.

Some kind of counter-clotting device which can cover artificial surfaces is urgently required. We can, of course, identify and synthesize powerful counter-clotting chemicals both inside and outside of the blood stream. The difficulty is to cover artificial parts with an absolutely permanent coating of such substances, either in the form of an artificial lamina or sheath, or more

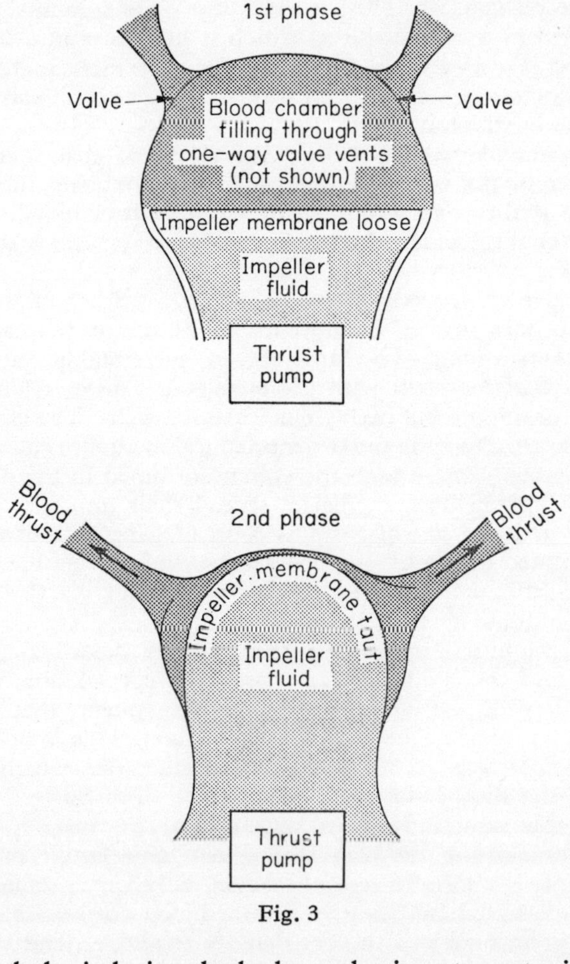

Fig. 3

intricately by inducing the body mechanisms to coat with their own anti-clotting substances those materials we introduce.

The heart pumps blood to oxygenate it. Currently there are two methods of oxygenating blood in external heart-lung machines, and it should be pointed out that by oxygenating is meant the treatment of blood by oxygen in a combination form, not by air. The principle of the treatment is the same in both methods, although from an engineering standpoint the methods themselves are very different.

The method that is most mechanical in the moving sense is the disc oxygenator. This consists of a plate spinning partially immersed in a bath of blood which it lifts clear in a fine film. Exposed in this way, violently and for a short time, the blood film absorbs oxygen, and falls back to change the consistency of the bath in which it spins.

The second method utilizes the principle that there is an exchange of gas to liquid when the gas is bubbled through it. Oxygen is therefore bubbled through a bath of blood, and the gas passes through the skin of the bubble to oxygenate the blood as it goes.

It is hardly necessary to point out that neither of these two ways has been chosen by nature for the exchanges that take place in the human lungs. The lungs are, in fact, a highly compressed tube exchange system with the air/blood transfer taking place by way of minute but highly efficient tube walls. The amount of blood exposed to air in the two mechanical methods is of necessity small by comparison with the volume of blood in the machine. But the human lung capillaries spread their lungfuls of blood over an area the size of a tennis court and, because of the very sophisticated design of their capillary walls, manage the transfer of huge amounts of oxygen, even though they get this oxygen only in a dilute air form.

Both the heart-lung designs that we have described, the disc dipper and the bubble maker, have one special disadvantage, which they do not share with any other system: that is, they present an interface between gas and blood. This is not a very obvious interface, in fact it is the molecular skin which, in the case of the disc, holds the blood to the disc. Surface tension creates this skin, and surface tension is really dynamic balance of forces existing between atmosphere and liquid pressures. Because it is a minute area of tension, only very minute things will be damaged by being in it. But blood corpuscles are just such minute things, with very delicate envelopes, and they can be ruptured and torn by the sudden forces that are involved in creating the surface skin.

Membrane oxygenators do not have this disadvantage. A membrane oxygenator is a very thin artificial skin which will pass oxygen from air on one side of it to blood on the other.

Ideally this system should not have any interfaces, that is, there should be no space left for air on the blood side of the membrane, while the blood itself should be in a tube or completely filled cavity.

Several membrane oxygenators have been designed recently. They employ various tough inert substances for their membranes, all of which are of exceptional thinness and all of which pass quite exceptional quantities of oxygen to blood, as well as stripping off some of the blood's surplus carbon dioxide. Unfortunately, efficient though they are they do not match up to the exchange capacity of living membrane.

There are ways however in which designers might push up the efficiency of such membrane systems. One way is to design a big multi-capillary as shown in Fig. 4, that is a large tube with

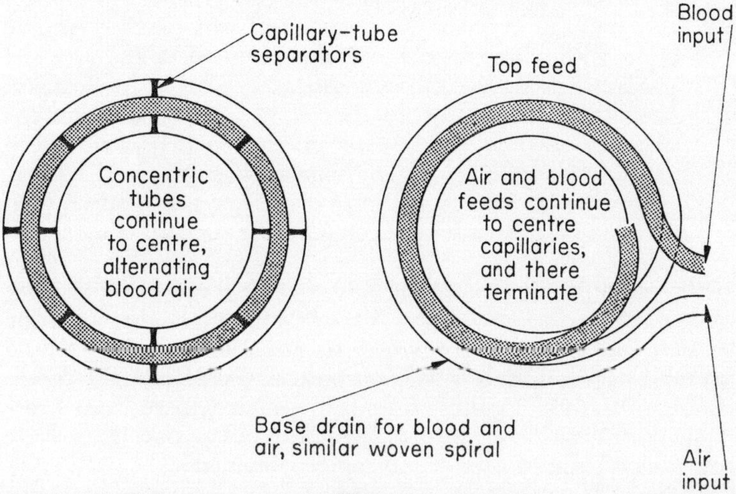

Fig. 4

hundreds of other tubes built within it, ranging down from those on the outside of the lung which are six inches in diameter to the centre ones, with a diameter of only 0·1 of a millimetre. Each of these tubes would be separated from the others by a gap only a fraction of a millimetre wide, and the separators keeping them apart would act as blood ducts, to organize the flow. Blood-flow and air-flow capillaries would alternate from core to circumference, producing a massive area of gas interchange surface within a small space.

Even with a design of this kind, however, the man-made lung

would still not gain the same area or efficiency as the human one. To overcome this problem, the designers might have to either:

a. Speed up the flow of blood through the capillary lung so that more blood would be oxygenated at a given surface for a given time. It ought to be remembered, though, that the delicacy of blood prevents its being forced against surfaces at too high a pressure.
b. Thin down the blood so that it flowed at a faster speed, and with less resistance. In this connection it should be pointed out that more and more is being discovered about the problems of thickening and thinning blood.
c. Arrange for blood essentials only to pass through the lung, bypassing blood components which are more or less passengers as far as oxygenation is concerned.
d. Combine all these three techniques, and possibly couple them with a fourth method, also essential to the artificial implant kidney, that of ionic assistance. This is the electrical propulsion through membranes of charged particles, and the selective blocking of others, a propulsion that could speed up the blood/oxygen interchange considerably. Of course, even when these chemical problems have been solved, man will still be left with very considerable surgical ones.

For example, as swallowing and speaking each involve very precise co-ordinations of air pressures and throat shapings, the two activities cannot be combined. Because both actions involve a common passage, no breath is permitted to pass into the throat when swallowing is going on and in speaking there is an overriding of the normal process of breathing out so that the precise pressures for sound production can be obtained.

These requirements are going to present very gross problems to heart-lung implant designers. It will be a very long time, for instance, before the kind of modifications of breathing that allow varied speech can be built into the heart-lung design. At best, for the foreseeable future the patient will be dependent on monotone, or near monotone, the expired air passing out of the throat in a steady stream, and producing a steady vocal tone.

As for swallowing, this may present even more difficult problems, because of back pressures down the throat, and it may well be that some kind of artificial reflex will have to be designed to cut out the air flow while food is passing. As for breathing in, it is likely that the air intakes of the lung pump will not be in the throat. As nostrils and throats are easily obstructed passages, it will be necessary to have a steady and unimpeded flow of air through an artificially opened vent in, say, the chest wall, or at the base of the neck.

In general, then, the problems of substituting human and mechanical grafts for natural lungs are theoretically understood, but practically it will be some time before they are realized. The same is not strictly true of kidney grafts, however, where there has been more success in both human and artificial experiments.

Kidney transplants were first carried out, as far as Europe is concerned, in 1959, and since that date some 1,400 people have received them. Originally the majority of kidneys for the transplants came from living donors, either parents or brothers or sisters of the patient, who donated one of their own organs for the purpose. But more recently the position has changed and now at least three-quarters of the transplanted kidneys are from corpses. The statistics of successful functioning of the grafted kidney, and of patient survival after the failure of the graft, are very interesting.

Grafts from different sources have very different chances of survival, as we can clearly see. Those from brothers and sisters come down to stabilize at about 70 per cent survival at 24 months. Parents do slightly worse, stabilizing at about 60 per cent, while corpses come a trailing third with just over 40 per cent.

There are several reasons for these differences, the most important being the relationship of the donor to the recipient, because its closeness determines the acceptability of the graft. We can see, in fact, that the blood tie makes a considerable difference. This is most clearly shown in the survival curve of corpse grafts, but it is also visible in the difference between those of brothers and sisters, who are more closely related to the patient, and parents. The closer the blood tie, in fact, the better the chance that the kidney will survive.

But there are several other factors which to some extent update these figures, and which have significant implications.

First, it seems that the chance of obtaining a blood-tie transplant is diminishing. The reason for this is not clear, but it is possible that surgeons are no longer pressing relatives to give organs. Secondly, there are very considerable differences in the degree of selection of grafts. It is of course much less easy to get what is known as a tissue-type test done on a corpse than on a living donor, yet the figures show that obtaining a good match is very important. Only 60 per cent of corpses were tissue-typed before a graft was taken from them, but getting a favourable tissue type means a 5 per cent increase in the rate of grafts that survive.

Simple statistics like these show that even relatively easy administrative procedures, like arranging for would-be donors to be tissue-typed before they die, may have very significant effects upon graft survival. Neither is there reason to doubt that more

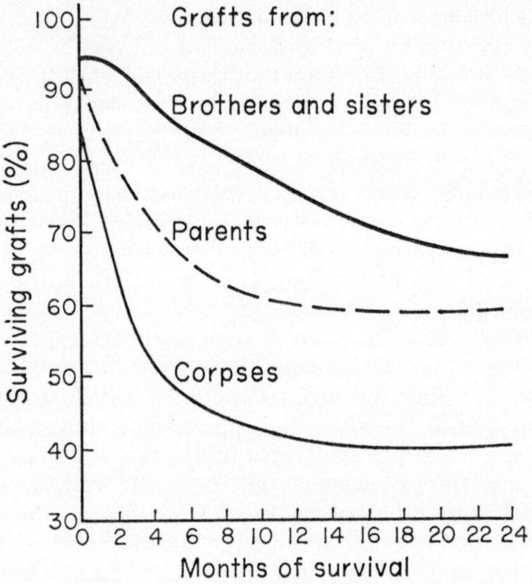

Fig. 5

sophisticated methods of combating rejection will have spectacular effects on the survival rate of kidney grafts.

The rejection of a graft does not of course automatically mean the death of the patient. Of those who suffer a rejection, approximately 60 per cent are taken on for intermittent dialysis, in other words their kidney function is maintained by a machine filter which washes their blood stream on a weekly basis. A smaller number can be given a second kidney transplant, when once again the familiar pattern of success or rejection, strongly influenced by the blood relationship, shows up in the figures.

Dialysis involves taking impure blood from the body, circulating it through a special form of extractor, and returning it to the body. Now if patients are to have regular treatments of one kind or another, whether these be the current ones of dialysis, etc., or the more speculative ones which we shall be discussing a little further on, there will be need for permanent access to the blood systems in the way of ports or shunts.

A shunt is a kind of miniaturized manhole, a connection made between an artery and a vein, which allows the blood supply to be tapped whenever the treatment is required. The installation of both ports and shunts is a delicate operation, and there is the added difficulty that the apparatus installed must not cause sepsis or discomfort by its presence. Ports made from Dacron, with a special skirt into which surrounding tissues can infiltrate, have proved highly successful. They are stoppered up much in the same way as are stoppers on air beds, but with greater hygiene. Shunts on the other hand, which involve attaching the miniaturized manhole to the patient's wrist and thus permitting direct access to a vein or artery, last only about six months, then have to be remade.

What is a kidney machine like? And since it seems that kidney donors are becoming scarcer, will it ever be possible to make an artificial implant organ?

The most important thing to note about modern kidney machines is that they are large, and most decidedly unportable and non-implantable. They usually consist of a mounted bed of permeable membranes made of plastic about four feet long and six inches thick through which the patient's blood is gradually filtered. Linked with this is the blood pumping, monitoring and fluid-giving unit, which ensures that a cleansing fluid is pumped through simultaneously with the blood, thus sucking off the unwanted products and clearing them away.

It is worth pointing out at this point that most modern kidney machines function at only about 50 to 70 per cent of their potential efficiency, and this is largely due to poor structural design. In order to equal the efficiency of human kidneys which are working full time, as it were, the kidney machine processes the patient's blood twice a week in twelve-hour shifts, separated by an interval of two or three days.

It is worth looking at the scale problems of an implant kidney with particular reference to the present size of external machines, and the way in which they are employed. Not only are they used on about a seventh of the number of cases that living kidneys are used, they are, as we have mentioned, only working at approximately 50 to 75 per cent of their optimum design efficiency. Therefore, allowing for peculiarities of scale, and the chance of their growing smaller as they become more efficient, there would appear to be the possibility of reducing them to ten or even twelve times their present size, providing they work continuously.

Now on this principle even the primitive renal dialyser which we have today could be brought down to the size of a large book, although the addition of the miniaturized pumping unit would double it. Of course, even at this size it would still be some five to ten times larger than the pair of natural kidneys it would replace, and of course it would have no power supply. But it is now within a workable dimension of reduction, instead of being quite outlandishly huge.

It is worth while asking why the artificial kidney is so large when the natural one is so small. The answer lies directly in the efficiency of the membranes through which the blood in both sorts of kidneys is perfused. The efficiency of natural membrane is very high, and that of artificial is very low, and consequently more artificial membrane is required to extract impurities from the blood than would be required for the same volume of blood passing through the natural kidney. Once more then, the success of an artificial implant organ seems to depend upon the development of a new sort of membrane. But if this is developed what will an implant artificial kidney be like?

Looking at the problem strictly from the dialysing standpoint (that is the leaching out of the blood of poisons like urea, uric acid and creatinine) we can visualize a capillary component, probably made of small tubes with a striking compactness. The problem of freshening up the dialysing fluids (that is cleaning the cleaner itself, and thus cutting down the amount of fluid required) may be handled by sorbents. Sorbents are materials which sop up the poisons which the dialyser has leached off, and render them harmless, or at least organize them in such a way that they can be disposed of.

For keeping the water balance of the blood steady, and to eliminate other poisonous substances that a capillary dialyser cannot tackle, a second filter stage would need to be added. This would be a very sophisticated filter indeed with a variable mesh, controlled and cleaned electrically, and capable of passing molecules of varied size, at varied rates. It would be monitored by probes in the blood supply, and represent the stage before the treated blood went back to the main stream.

The implant artificial kidney would require powering up, of course, beyond the demands of natural kidneys. It would need a small pump for the capillary section and the secondary filter, a steady current potential for the electrical diffuser, and outlets to dispose of the debris. None of these surgical and engineering problems would be easy, but big though they are they do not approach those involved in transplanting livers or brains.

With the liver we have a situation not unlike that presented by the lung transplant attempts. Although the results in animals are surprisingly good, those in human beings do not reach these standards. In fact, of about forty patients who have received liver grafts, there are probably only a dozen patients who have survived more than a year. When the operation is done on dogs, however, there is a good chance that the liver will take: dogs which were grafted in 1964 are still surviving.

Most informed opinion seems to settle once again on two main causes for this great mortality in humans. The first fixes on the problems of preserving the graft liver, which is usually taken from a corpse, and the second on the very difficult surgical pre-graft procedures, which may occupy valuable hours before the actual operation begins. It is known, for example, that if a liver is not under very strict preservation control for some time before the donor's death it may be irretrievably damaged. Such control may be impossible with a dying patient, as indeed may be the vital early surgical intervention to ease the transfer.

Another very difficult hurdle is the patient's response to immunosuppressive drugs, designed to stop the liver being rejected. It is now known that the liver is a valuable ally in curbing rejection (in cases where other organs are grafted), but it cannot cope with its own rejection.

Many of the same problems also apply to brains. When we think about transplantation of the human brain, we must compartmentalize our thoughts somewhat. There are really two broad problems involved, the first being the transfer of brain tissue from one brain to another and its maintenance as a physiological entity when the transplant is complete. The other encroaches on mind and identity because it raises the whole issue of nerve-cell reconnection, in other words the combination in an electrical sense of brain with brain. Of these two problems the first is by far the easiest to understand and speculate upon, because it involves experimental work which has already been done on dog brains.

Dog-brain transplants involve a vast amount of preparatory work in reorganizing the circulation of a section of the brain so that it can be effectively coupled up to a single artery when it is transplanted. It is not, in fact, transferred to a recipient dog's brain. Rejection is not an issue in brain transplants because brain tissues are quite compatible even when alien to each other. Instead, because of the coupling-up problems, it is replaced in the subject's own neck, in a small pouch of skin. Close monitoring after the transplant shows that it functions quite well as a physical entity, though of course it does not control anything in the subject's body.

The transplanting of livers and brains has as yet no theoretical basis, let alone any practical designs or attempts. Both these organs, however, consist of non-dividing or slowly dividing cells, and it is just possible that a very comprehensive cellular transplant system will be developed which will involve the diffusion of all organs composed of non-dividing or slowly dividing cells (bone marrow would therefore be excluded) with replacements for defectives and aberrants.

And now, as we have seen, the immunological transplant barrier weakens between closely related persons – in identical twins vanishes altogether. The technique of comprehensive cell transplantation, then, must be to create banks of cells with twin compatibility – in other words to grow another parallel individual, strictly for the purposes of cell transfer.

Experimental cultures of embryonic material have been developed from the sperm and ova of animals without cross-fertilization. This technique (known as experimental parthenogenesis) could be greatly expanded. With it might come the possibility of developing parallel banks of parthenogenetic material for every person, consisting of replacement cells for vulnerable and otherwise irreplaceable organs.

The greatest difficulty would probably come in ensuring that cells penetrated their target organ (a much lesser difficulty would be ensuring that they knew their role when they arrived – experiments already show that they do). The problems of targeting and clustering round the failing organ would be relatively simple, but the gaining of entry through a mass of crosslinked connective tissue quite another. It is virtually certain then that some vigorous method of breaking down crosslink material would be necessary before the replacement cells could gain admittance. And this, of course, takes us on to some of the anti-crosslinking devices to be discussed in a later section.

We have discussed some very drastic modifications of man, within a range of speculative procedures. Let us, as a conclusion, deal with some of the simpler and more immediately feasible sorts of transplant, which may themselves become very important in extending lifespans.

Tissue typing (the matching of lymphocyte/leucocyte attack characteristics, so that they cancel each other out) is steadily becoming more sophisticated. By careful cultivation of tissues and serums from graft donors and would-be recipients, and by consequent composition of a list of characteristics relating to the antigens which cultivation exposes, lists of compatible and incompatible items can be drawn up, and best fittings of items sought.

Looking at the problem from another angle, biologists have assumed that if a skin graft from an unrelated donor to a recipient survives twenty or more days without the use of a rejection suppression drug, then any kind of organ graft between this pair will survive permanently, when drugs are given. In fact, the chances of this kind of skin-graft survival taking place are one in thirty. One in thirty is about 3 per cent, and therefore if we were considering linking prospective graftees together long before it was necessary for them to consider giving or accepting grafts we would have to perform a large number of skin grafts before we hit on a mutual pair.

But let us conceive a situation where miniaturized skin grafting becomes a reality, and it is possible to perform a hundred tiny skin grafts within a small patch of skin. If the hundred grafts were randomly taken, then it might be possible subsequently to identify 3 per cent of the survivors twenty or more days later. In this way, and very speedily, large numbers of highly compatible graftees could be linked administratively, and might undertake to mutually donate organs to each other in case of need. In fact, the techniques to perform this feat are in process of development. Already very minute skin graftings have been performed in mice; and ways of subsequently locating them perfected. What is required therefore is a method of multiple grafting, separation, mingling and subsequent application.

One kind of transplantation which could be regarded as intermediate therapy, but which nevertheless has at present a significant part to play in the treatment of burns, is temporary skin grafting. We know that only a very small percentage of skin grafts between unrelated donors stay on their transplant sites longer than twenty-one days. However a large proportion will hold for between nine and fourteen days – a feature that is most useful in the cases of burn victims. Burned people lose fluids at an enormous rate, and develop various forms of poisoning because of their lack of skin protection. If unselected skin from a skin bank is grafted on to their burns, it seals up the weeping areas and cuts down the risk of infection. Eventually it sloughs off, but not before it has given the patient valuable time. But time for what?

If we establish a dispersed graft bank which can call up compatible donors to give, in the case of skin graft, a small piece of skin each, to patch a big burn, then at least ten days would be required to gather up all these donors, obtain their grafts, and collect all the fragments together for the full transplant. These ten days could be bought by intermediate grafts, leaving the patient strong enough to take the compatible tissue at the end of that time.

Finally, let us consider a field which in graft terms might be regarded as the simplest of all. There are several areas of the human body (and not only of the human body) that do not seem to have reject sensitivity, that is to say, transplants from incompatible donors do not trip off the usual violent rejection reactions that are found with other areas. The range of such organs is somewhat curious. It includes, as previously mentioned, the brain (which at the moment is no great help), the testis (there are no records as yet of sex organ grafts, but they may be in the offing), the eye and the bone marrow. These last two offer a narrow but useful salient of graft possibilities, free from the danger of rejection.

For example, when bone marrow has succumbed to an overdose of radiation, its death cuts down the body's blood substances, and soon leads on to anaemia. Bone marrow cellular injections from unrelated donors have saved the marrows, and probably the lives, of people receiving lethal doses of radiation. As has been mentioned in another chapter, marrow cells multiply at a colossal speed, and soon fill up and crowd out damaged or dead inmates, a phenomenon which assists the injection process.

Eye transplantation offers an even more useful avenue in the form of corneal grafts, which have given vision back to thousands of blind persons. However neither of these two openings offer much scope for extended lifespans. Eyes are invaluable, but not vital, and bone marrow, provided it does not become radiated, seems to be immortal, since, as far as modern analysis goes, the cells of young and old marrows show no ageing differences.

This then is the state of play as far as transplants are concerned. Certain natural organs can be grafted with great success, others with less, and some with almost none at all. At the same time sources of graft supply seem to be diminishing, and indeed it now seems that supply has never been organized, nor could ever be organized, to meet a mass demand, since the difficulties with the preservation of grafts must necessarily eliminate large amounts of available graft material.

At the same time artificial grafts in the shape of implanted organs are in slow process of development, particularly slow when the organ involves moving parts, or needs big quantities of power to run it. Materials, their reliability and their efficiency also pose huge problems to the designer of artificial organs, problems which perhaps must wait for the 'spin-off' results of other, non-related technical achievements.

3

The Engineer Intervenes

As man strives for an extended lifespan, and perhaps immortality, he will see a group of problems which lie within the scope of the engineer. These will present themselves because the body is a dynamic organism, built to move about, and have components move within it in various hydraulic, pneumatic and electromagnetic ways. Such movements with their consequences are essentially engineering ideas, and even at this early stage we can identify two main ways in which this expert will be able to extend lifespans.

1. He will be able to identify likely sites of mechanical failure within the body, so that preventive action can be taken in advance of catastrophe.
2. He will suggest methods whereby the deterioration chains of the body may be interrupted or diverted.

Now nowhere is the influence likely to be more felt than in the body's harder structures, which develop slowly, regenerate, if they do at all, with difficulty, bear heavy stresses, and use as building materials inorganic substances of various kinds, to make themselves rock hard and resilient.

Cartilages, bones and teeth are such structures, which is not the same as saying that they share all those characteristics in common (they do not) but which identifies them as being in a special category of mechanical risk, and thus of special interest to the engineer.

Cartilage, the slippery sheathing material of joints, is, for example, a unique substance in the body. It is entirely lacking in blood vessels, yet it sustains itself in a situation of tremendous stress by a system of sponging up nutrients from its own lubricating fluids. It is in the front line of the battle of wear and tear, and yet engineers do not understand how it manages to keep itself from being worn out in a week let alone a lifetime. But incredibly competent though it is, it does fail.

Degenerative Arthritis (Joint Breakdown)

One of the most important causes of weakening in the skeleton is degenerative arthritis, a breakdown of the smooth cartilage surfaces which allow the bones to touch and rub together with minimum friction. Although the condition is easily diagnosible, and almost everybody suffers from it, there is still controversy over its exact nature. The problem is that there seem to be two diseases, a mild degenerative roughening of certain areas of a joint, starting in early maturity and steadily progressing until in old age the joint moves with some difficulty but still moves, and a second, much rarer, much more savage breakdown of cartilage tissue, generally occurring in old age and usually making the joint immobile.

There is a relationship between these two kinds of degeneration. For instance, there is evidence that joints that most commonly show mild degenerative changes in youth and middle age are those which most commonly develop the savage breakdowns of old age. But many old people do not develop the serious ailment, which suggests that although they have degenerative tendencies these are in some way prevented from progressing to a severely disabling stage.

It is not, of course, unusual to have ailments of different origins affecting the same organ. But despite this, and the curious paradox that the mild degenerative disease begins in areas which do not bear much actual joint stress, while the severer arthritis affects parts carrying great loads, there is some vague evidence that the two diseases have a common origin, or are part of the same process.

The mild joint deterioration begins in areas of joints which are carrying very little weight, because the body anatomy has so developed as to exclude them from work except under unusual contortions of the limb. It probably starts because cartilage which is not used cannot get an adequate supply of nourishment, such nourishment being absorbed from the joint lubricant because of pummelling from the top. Such mild degeneration is perfectly harmless, and may remain so, except in cases where because of a variety of circumstances it extends into the no-man's-land which separates the low-pressure areas from those with high pressure. If it weakens the cartilage there and, because of unusual movement or for any other reason is forced to take a heavy load, then a break may occur and an ulcer form.

Once an ulcer has formed, even though it is marginal to the high-pressure area, a joint catastrophe may follow. The surface of a cartilage, being built up out of layers of fibres arranged in a criss-cross pattern, is designed to resist splitting. Its structure gives great strength under stress and strain, but allows an ulcer to develop a fault in different directions at different layers. An ulcer on the margin then has a good prospect of growth, and the more it infiltrates the high-pressure region, the better its prospects become because there the split fibres are under greater stress.

Many people escape ulceration, and many ulcers do not extend. But, of course, present life may well be too short to demonstrate what might happen in extended lifespans – given enough joint play, or accidents. Perhaps the two diseases seem to be different, but this is only because normal lifespans do not give them enough scope to become one.

The present attempts to solve the problems of arthritic joints are almost entirely confined either to the design and installation of artificial joints (usually the hip joint) or the selection and grafting of natural joints (taken from cadavers). As to the former, experience has narrowed down the range of materials and combinations to an almost exclusive use of metal balls and sockets, or metal to high-density polyethylene combinations as substitutes for the natural hipbone/pelvis joint. Within limits there are now effective substitutes – the important word being 'limits'. Such joints are not offered to hikers, cross-country runners, dustmen or weight lifters, in other words they provide an incomplete substitution. They tend to be fitted to quiet sedentary people with the prospect of short careful lives. Even under these circumstances they show wear, and acceptance problems related to the metal of the joints and the cements which fix them to the natural bone. The Russians, on the other hand, have been experimenting with joint grafts. These involve the grafting, in place of diseased joints, of complete joints together with sections of supporting bone taken from corpses.

As far as is known these bone/joint grafts have been fairly successful. It is an accepted fact that bone grafts, even homografts (those using bone from another body) are much more likely to knit than homograft soft-tissue organs such as kidneys and hearts. The reason is probably that in a bone homograft the body fragment transferred is not truly autonomous, in other words it is not an organ complete with systems but a matrix into which the host systems can infiltrate and wind. Getting rid of something when one is deeply involved in it is always a problem, and this means that rejection here is much less likely.

But bone/joint grafts are not likely to provide an answer to the arthritis of extended lifespans. To begin with the mass grafting of joints would soon exhaust stocks from corpses, always supposing that in a successful 'halt' situation there would be any corpses. Animals might be bred for joint grafting, of course. The problem here is that animals with joints big enough to stand the weight of man would be anatomically different from him, and the grafts they provided might need much modification. In any case there is a much more obvious and wider reason why we should not consider metal joints or grafts as likely future techniques. Both require extensive surgery, and both demand a great deal of mental and physical resilience from would-be seekers of relief. If extended lifespans are to be worth living they will need to be free from the prospects of intermittent surgery (however sophisticated), and all techniques which maintain the indefinite life will have to be painless, convenient and if possible self maintaining.

With such criteria in mind how might the speculative engineer approach this problem?

Let us conceive of a new, immensely sophisticated material, organic or inorganic, but possessed of one overriding capability, that of combining with cartilage in a minimally intensive way. This new material might be injected into the body to form a reservoir which could be drawn upon as required. Immediately the first signs of degenerative arthritis appeared at the joints the material would move to fill and smooth over the fissures. The greater the deterioration, the greater would be the substitution, the deeper the fissure effect, the deeper would be the penetration of the material.

The effect of such a comprehensive replacement could be to nullify the effects of both forms of osteoarthritis, since in the event of the two diseases not in fact being stages of one process, cartilage failure within the pressure area would be dealt with in the same substitutional way.

The completely resurfaced joint or joints would, of course,

be bonded on to underlying bone bases, and no longer dependent upon the efficiency of support systems to keep them smooth and slippery. They would however be very much dependent upon the continued strength and resilience of this underlying bone, in other words a resurfacing technique would need a perfect guarantee of the absence of osteoporosis for permanent success, a requirement that we shall examine shortly. This aside, for the moment we can draw up a specification for the superplastic.

First, of course, it will have to be specific in its attraction for joint cartilage; any generalizing, in other words bonding itself to surfaces other than cartilage, might be disastrous. Then it must be capable of a high degree of self-lubrication (since the natural joint-lubrication systems are probably adaptable only to natural cartilage, and may not serve a new material properly). It would of course be an immense advantage if the material could mimic the cartilage structure absolutely, filling in a precise matrix in the process. Then, because this would minimize wear it would of course need to be an absolutely stable and predictable material, not giving off toxins or allowing itself to be dispersed. Its rate of wear would have to be known very precisely so that new infusions could be given whenever it was known that wear had occurred. As to wear itself, it is quite likely that a definite mechanical advantage would be available in so far as the artificial joint would have the exact contours of the original. And finally, of course, it would have to be cheap, and easy to administer – not taking up much time, or putting the patient into shock or side effects.

The actual mechanisms of depositing the superplastic on to the joint surfaces could well be very complex. If, for example, the relationship between the existing cartilage and the superplastic were a sophisticated one, it might be possible for remodelling to take place with no more than local control, in other words, after the superplastic had remodelled itself to the original joint dimensions no more deposition would take place, regardless of how much superplastic were floating about in the blood stream. On the other hand, if no such sophisticated relationship were developed, only enough superplastic to repair a calculated erosion would be allowed to circulate. In such circumstances it would be necessary, indeed it might be vital, to have very exact measurements of the extent to which a specific joint had been eroded. Sufficient superplastic could then be liberated to coat that joint only, without excess.

From the very beginning of the sequel of replacement the

superplastic would, of course, start to wear. In this it would be imitating the experiences of natural cartilage, which itself suffers slow abrasions, owing to the imperfections of the lubricating system. There would be one significant difference, however; for whereas the debris that falls from a wearing joint of natural cartilage is swiftly absorbed by the body (provided it is not in the form of actual bone granules) that which rubbed from the superplastic joint would be by definition insoluble. Here the material's designers would face the paradox of having to produce a material, impregnable while acting as a joint, but swiftly disposable as debris.

If the paradox could not be resolved, the consequences would significantly affect the efficiency of treated joints. Debris and sludge would gradually collect in the sumps of the joints, and eventually interfere with the flexibility of joints' motion, or set up gross inflammation.

Another feature of the replacement process which might cause difficulty would be the likelihood that the substitution would not occur evenly in terms of either space or time. By this I mean that at one and the same instant a joint might consist of natural cartilage and superplastic deposit, both wearing at different rates, and both requiring replacement with the same substance. Of course this would only be an interim problem, since eventually all the natural cartilage would disappear, thus offering a truly homogeneous material for self-maintenance. But while the changeover lasted, it might give rise to very real difficulties, particularly if the relationship between cartilage and plastic, and plastic and plastic, were an unsophisticated one, as hinted at in the previous sections.

There are several ideas in this programme which may seem somewhat wild, unless one is in possession of some knowledge of advanced medicine. Although it is true that there has been rather poor success with experiments to graft artificial material to natural tissue outside the hard structure ventures like metal shafts to bone, there are three advances which have a kind of optimistic relevance to the problem of superplastics.

The first is that an adhesive has recently been perfected which will stick blood vessels together, thus clearing the difficulty of bonding soft substances in the body. Secondly, a very great deal of work has been done in making substances specific in locating different organs or cells. Thirdly, much is already known about the basic constituents of cartilage; research has shown that far from being a very complex substance, it is principally composed of a kitchen ingredient – gelatine.

But, of course, success in the long term would undoubtedly depend upon the continuing strength of the underlying bone base, and the continuing absence of osteoporosis.

Osteoporosis (Bone Weakening)

Before we gain insight into the mechanisms of bone weakening, we have to know something about the way in which bones keep their strength – while they keep it. The skeletal system is too intricate to describe in great detail, but briefly the growth and maintenance sequences seem to work in this way.

The vital component in the system is the builder bone cell, the osteoblast. But just as the osteoblast has the task of bone building, it may also, having undergone certain vital transformations, destroy bone. In both sorts of bone, at all life stages, and even in the very unbonelike beginnings of bone, when the young organism is developing, the builder bone cell sets about its task commanded by some as yet only dimly understood chemical in the blood current near it. Having previously lined itself up appropriately with other osteoblasts, the builder bone cell starts to build a frame or matrix round itself using as building materials various highly concentrated nutrients again transported to it along the blood stream. This frame is at first elastic, but by mechanisms as yet imperfectly understood it rapidly becomes rigid. It undergoes this transformation as a result of a process of mineralization, in other words little by little it is turned into a hard rocky structure with crystals of calcium and phosphates stiffening up the hitherto flexible gum-like frame.

The next stage in the process is, according to one theory, perhaps the obvious consequence for the osteoblast, for having busily built a frame around itself, and quite literally bricked itself in, it becomes immobilized. Immobilized but not impotent – in fact very potent indeed, for remaining walled up in its own matrix it is in an excellent position to reverse the whole process of bone construction and bring the whole bone house crashing down.

It is renamed as a result of being immobilized, being now dubbed an osteocyte. Osteocytes keep close links with osteoblasts and indeed are held to organize the other phase of a continuous process of bone formation and reabsorption. Bones are not once and for all entities but, particularly in growing adolescents, are kept up to changing specification by a constant process of remodelling. Bone formation and reabsorption form essential parts of this remodelling process.

When maturity is reached, a plateau or balance between bone formation and absorption is reached, in other words just as much bone is being laid down as demolished. But shortly after maturity the balance tilts to demolition, particularly for women, and from then on, with pauses, of course, for the process is not a continuous decline, bones become lighter and weaker.

The osteocyte is held to play a vital part in this decline, although the mechanisms of its role in normal degeneration are not by any means understood. It seems to have the capability of giving off a very powerful chemical solvent which attacks its surrounding frame, dissolves it and, of course, causes a collapse of the minerals which have crystallized on to it. Both frame and crystals swill away in body fluids, the bone becomes less dense, and weakens.

Something triggers the osteocyte to do this, and that something is not easy to detect. When people are kept in bed for a long time, their bones do become lighter and weaker, and in such cases (seemingly an acceleration of the normal ageing process) the inactivity of their muscles causes some change in the blood supply, which acts as a trigger mechanism. However, osteoporosis goes on minutely, but steadily, even when an ageing person's limbs are fully mobile. It is possible then that something else, perhaps another kind of blood change, which is continuously operative, can have the same triggering effect as immobility.

Unfortunately this is only one side of the osteoporosis problem; for the disease also occurs in situations outside the normal ageing process, and not associated with immobility.

Women develop it after the menopause; vitamin deficiencies can trigger it off, and so can the indiscriminate administration of drugs like cortisone. We have therefore to face a range of possibilities as to its cause.

First, there could be several different ways in which the osteocyte might be affected, all different, and brought about by differing influences, but all equally efficient at making the osteocyte start to break the matrix down. Secondly, there could be a single final cause, say a chemical change in the blood, brought about by vitamin deficiencies, immobility, drug influences, etc., either singly or in contribution.

Recently a new technique has been developed for the manufacture of a sponge metal. The matrix of this sponge is a plastic, and after being impregnated with metal, it is burned out systematically leaving only the metal behind. This is a current example of the way in which a weak matrix can be used to create a strong structure, and then discarded without detriment to the residual structure.

Now if a new crystalline material could be designed, with an exceptional resistance to being dissolved, and were to be preferred by the body systems for hardening up the matrix rather than natural bone-toughening minerals, then it might not matter how much osteocytic activity took place. The osteocytes could work themselves up into an osteoporotic frenzy without disturbing the mineralization.

The matrix, of course, might disappear entirely, but this would not affect the indissoluble mineral, which would lose no significant strength by its departure. Such a structure might, of course, become very difficult to manage if it ever fractured. But conceivably it could be so designed that it would never fracture.

One very serious problem with such an indestructible bone coral might be weight. The mineral, possibly a synthesized mineral/metal might be denser *in situ* than normal bone and therefore heavier. A marginal increase might not matter – bones after all are not the heaviest component of the body – but if, for example, the bone coral were to double or treble the normal weight, then matters might be very different. The musculature and its circulating system are built to cope with reasonably wide tolerances in terms of overall body weight, but there are, of course, limits, and if these were exceeded, a whole new range of problems would emerge. It is also possible, of course, to speculate upon various compensating techniques which would enable the body to cope adequately with increased loads. The basic problem is one of transport, and the capacity of the circulatory system to carry muscle nutrients, and disperse muscle wastes, and we may be able to develop the transport system substantially, and make it carry more for a given unit of flow.

Neither is weight the only possible problem. Another is timing – judging the appropriate point to start the new crystallizing process – and timing here does depend on the extent to which the bones need to be remodelled.

Remodelling forms an essential part of the processes of bone growth. This involves demineralizing, remineralizing and all the other complex processes that allow youthful bones to lengthen, and not to lose strength in the lengthening. Remodelling is probably a total process with all parts of the growing bone involved, and while it goes on no attempt can be made to fix the mineral content of bone, because this might interfere with growth.

Once growth had ceased, however, substitution could begin.

It would not need to be a lifelong process. The actual mineral turnover, apart from in some deep areas, is very swift, and within a decade therefore a majority of crystals could be changed from destructible to indestructible forms. If the idea of indestructibility seems strange, it should be remembered that fluoride, taken up by the body as a tooth decay preventive, has already been found to be indestructible and remains *in situ* indefinitely.

There is no doubt that in normal bone the mineral and the matrix together constitute a most resilient combination; one which shows great resistance to cracking, and is capable of withstanding enormous strains whether these be of compression or of tension. But it is probable that if the mineral could not be washed out, and were to become a permanent fixture, it would in the absence of the flexible matrix form a very rigid material, with a good deal of compression resistance, but little toughness. This would pose considerable problems, because bones must be capable of different sorts of stress resistance, and brittleness might seriously limit the usefulness of the limbs.

This is where a very advanced materials technology might be able to come up with a solution. At present much research is concentrating on the problem of creating new, rather than adapting old, materials for modern uses. But this could be but a phase, and research might find ways of reorganizing the internal molecular structure of a substance in a way that would make it tolerate a great range of stresses.

Bones as it happens do things other than just provide a frame for the softer structures. For example, they are used as reservoir to keep up the calcium balance of the body; they act as calcium current accounts which are constantly being drawn upon, and credited. Any attempt, therefore, to make the bone/mineral content permanent, which locked up such calcium deposits, would be dangerous, and it would be necessary to reserve certain parts of bones to keep up the in and out transfer of vital chemicals. Whether such reservations would act as focuses for ageing must remain speculative; much would depend probably on other systems continuing to make demands for calcium.

The consequences of osteoporosis are very serious. Bones do not behave under stress like other solids which have a continuous crystalline structure. Such substances as metal or plastic may crack under stress, the split spreading into the material, gradually picking up support as it goes from the internal dynamics of the system, until finally it leaps forward at a phenomenal speed to make a complete fracture. Materials like metals and plastics are relatively impotent in these circumstances. They do not normally have methods of deflecting the crack, and absorbing its strength. They also cannot shift crack resistance about internally to make it difficult for splits to start.

Bones, on the other hand, can do these things. They have been cunningly designed to make it very difficult for stresses to convert themselves easily into progressive splittings. They toughen up in anticipation of compression and strain, and seal up cracks in the rear of a crack tip, always supposing that they have allowed the crack to develop in the first place.

Osteoporosis destroys the resilience of these systems. It tends to have its maximum effect in areas where the bone has to take the maximum strain, and it is likely to be most severe at an age when a person's balance is most precarious, thus increasing the risk of fall and fracture. In fact, the coming together of such factors as loss of muscle power, impairment of sense of equilibrium, declining vision and poor hearing, coupled with the gradually increasing menace of osteoporosis, makes fractures, especially of the hip joint, one of the most likely causes of death amongst aged people. The fracture itself is not generally the direct cause of death, however – it is the immobility that results from it. A person's mobility seems to be vital at all ages and desperately so in old age, when enforced immobility can cause pressure sores, or a form of pneumonia, or various other lethal ailments.

Because of the complexity implied by this picture, it is clear that eliminating osteoporosis is not likely to be a simple task. It might therefore conceivably be more rational to concentrate upon ways in which the process could be neutralized in its effects. Fortunately there are some pointers to how this might be done.

Crystals of phosphate and calcium are much in use in the body. As well as providing the stiffening element in bone they also form the basic constituents of teeth, although in teeth they are packed much tighter, and their matrix is much more fragile.

If man does become a self-maintaining machine in the sense of being able to sustain a complete cell replacement in soft tissues, then his teeth will need to be a great deal more durable than they are at present. It is also probably significant that nobody who is engaged in avant-garde dentistry is much concerned with the development of dentures. False teeth, in the sense of artificial teeth pegged to a plate, are a grotesquely inadequate method of helping at the eating process, being insanitary, inconvenient, and prone to mechanical failure. An extended lifetime with dentures would be a nightmare, and since one of the objects of living long is to enjoy life, they are not likely to play an important future role. Faced in fact with the speculation of a five-hundred-year life span, the research-directed dental surgeon thinks first of four main causes of tooth deterioration: decay, abrasions, periodontal disease, and accidental injuries. Dental decay seems to be caused by acid-producing bacteria attacking the inorganic crystals forming the enamel of the tooth. The crystals themselves are very vulnerable to such acid and once weakened or destroyed, the whole matrix of the tooth starts to come apart at the seams, cracks spread, harder layers detach, and the tooth substance begins to rub away quickly.

Now, if the bacteria which have been isolated can be cultured, and will yield a vaccine which gives an immunity, a whole range of dental problems will be solved. Anti-decay vaccination would seem then to be the most promising long-term solution to decay,* although fluoridation may well be tried as a short-term approach if the political difficulties surrounding it can be resolved. Unfortunately, however, the elimination of decay does not of itself generate indefinite tooth life: the threats of abrasion, periodontal disease and tooth injuries still remain.

This abrasion or rubbing down of teeth is a lifelong process, the disastrous results of which can often be seen in patients as 'young' as the fifth decade of life. Principally it occurs because we bite and grind our food, which contains a minute but significant quantity of abrasives, either picked up like dust in the course of preparation, or actually part of the food itself. We also brush our teeth, or some of us do, twice a day, with soft abrasive pastes. A minority, especially those with poorly meshing teeth, or suffering from tensions, grind by night while asleep. All these abrasive processes take the toll of the dental surfaces, so that a man, in spite of being resistant to decay, given a five-hundred-year life span might still be left with no teeth at all by his twentieth decade, because the normal process of wear had ground them down to stumps.

* Acidogenic theory:

(1) Lactic bacteria such as Streptococcus mutans feed on sucrose from ingested food.

(2) A glutinous bacterial plaque is formed on the surface of the teeth and the extra-cellular polysaccharide from the sugars keeps up a supply of food to the lactic bacteria.

(3) Bacteria produce acid which dissolves hydroxyapatite crystals (enamel).

Faced with this very difficult problem the research-directed dental surgeon suggests three possible approaches – sheathing, implanting, and regenerating. In principle, sheathing involves covering the teeth with an ultra hard, abrasion-resisting, plastic substance (preferably five times more resistant to rubbing than dental enamel) which can be swiftly moulded, and immovably bonded to the patient's own teeth.

Unfortunately, although very tough substances, both natural (like jade) and artificial (like carborundum) are in existence, and much more sophisticated syntheses of ceramics and metals are being tried out, such materials, new or old, are very difficult to handle. They do not mould easily (an essential feature of any mass resheathing process) and they do not stick reliably. And mass resheathing with reliable sticking would certainly be necessary if very long lifespans became common.

Materials lacking, it is certainly possible, though we must make several more assumptions. For the treatment to be done on a mass basis we must assume a very sophisticated moulding device, capable of taking impressions from both jaws, which will perform two command functions. First, it would decide if the mesh of the original teeth were the best obtainable, having regard to the geometry of the jaws. Then it would 'remember' or reconstruct this mesh for a two-jaw sheath mould, and command the action of a second, very sophisticated device, perhaps a sandblasting, ultrasonic, high-speed turbine diamond, or even a laser cutting machine which would shave off the surfaces of the anaesthetized patient's existing teeth. Finally, it would master-mind the bonding of the new dental sheaths to the existing tooth roots, test each individual tooth for bonding and the whole mesh of the jaws for fit.

Of course, there might be certain additional problems springing from the altered mesh of the teeth, or even from the fact that the original profile had been reproduced exactly, but artificially. Chief amongst these might be problems of tongue and cheek biting, resulting from the mouth's muscle tone being disturbed. We ought not to imagine, however, that with advanced psychological conditioning techniques these kind of problems could not be solved.

Implanting

The second field of speculation is implanting. Implants (experimentally they have already been tried) involve the pegging of artificial or natural teeth directly to the jawbone. Taking a long view this seems a promising, even perhaps an essential, technique because with the torque of time natural tooth roots overlaid with sheaths might start to rock about on their rootings. Very hard artificial teeth, screwed or riveted to the jawbones, would certainly give a firmer and more durable foundation for lifespans extending thirty or forty decades.

However, there are problems. Although jawbones will take artificial teeth, provided they are not made from substances with an organic content, the circle of gum tissue surrounding them is precarious, and inflammation is common around the upper roots. What is still needed is the development of a speedily permeable artificial tooth, which the gum tissue can infiltrate in much the same way as creeper winds itself into a trellis. A tooth of this kind would be a much more durable possibility, but if it were to be developed it would highlight the problem of actually arranging for the mass implantings of the jaws of millions of patients in extended lifespans.

Requiring extractions for such new implants would be psychologically unacceptable, and economically impracticable. An essential supplementary development might be a substance, possibly akin to a hormone in its action, to stimulate tooth loosening, and to precipitate what we might call a 'tooth moult'. This hormone-like substance might be administered to patients a short time before they attended for their implant sets. Provided all went well, the patients' natural teeth could be extracted, perhaps by finger pull, thus clearing both jaws for a swift automated implanting session. A breakthrough in dental anaesthetics which allowed a deep local aneasthesia to be obtained from a spray would ease these sessions considerably.

Regenerations

This very speculative notion of a tooth moult is important in the third, possibly the most sophisticated, and certainly very much the most appealing of advanced dental techniques – regenerations. At man's present stage of evolution he grows only two sets of teeth in one lifetime. And yet there is no theoretical reason why he should not be able to grow many more. The actual process is not biologically complex, and certainly not debilitating, but the problem is that reseeding of teeth does not, in fact, occur again after the milk teeth drop out, and the second teeth emerge.

But if a controlled reseeding could be triggered at a hormonal command, then a man could have a new set of teeth to replace a worn one as soon as there was sufficient wear to cause pain or interfere with his eating. Such a 'tooth moult' would have to be a comprehensive shedding, because a patchy programme with some teeth in eruption, and others dropping out, would play havoc with eating. The best sequence, if tooth development could be speeded up, might be:

first – a comprehensive 'tooth moult', with a complete clearance of the mouth in a matter of days, and an absolute minimum of 'loosening' time.
second – the reseeding process with a very fast growth.
third – a temporary denture set to carry the patient through the regeneration period.

These three speculative techniques, sheathing, implanting and regenerating, may seem very advanced by correct standards of dental care, but in fact some of the basic research to convert them from fantasies to actualities is already in hand.

Unfortunately the same cannot be said for the third important factor of tooth deterioration – periodontal disease. This disease causes loosening of teeth by the action of bacterial poisons on the attachment of the gums. It is a similar process to the formation of the crystal-destroying acids mentioned previously, but the objectives and effects differ. The action of the poisons is insidious but in the end devastating: the gum strips from the teeth and the bone of root and jaw recedes.

Again there are three ways in which research and development may in the end be capable of defeating periodontal disease. First, it may be possible to cause a genetic alteration in the development of the collagen element in the gum tissue. Collagen is ostensibly a tough substance but it has a peculiar vulnerability to bacterial attack. However, by intervening decisively in the way in which it is made, it may be possible to make it very resistant to poisons produced by bacteria.

A second method may be to grow new gum. At present the regeneration of gums after periodontal disease is something beyond the capabilities of the body. But regenerative techniques (which may also include other seemingly killable body structures) may permit new growth on old structural stock.

And finally but very speculatively, because one is looking for comprehensive rather than patchwork techniques, there is gum grafting. But this, although theoretically possible now, is unpromising, because of the difficulties of obtaining reliable supplies of gum for grafting, and because of the high degree of manipulative skill required for what might prove to be a mass demand operation.

So now we come to the last of the great dental threats, damage to teeth from injuries. It is highly likely that during very long lifespans teeth will be broken by such happenings as blows or falls or industrial accidents. However, the artificial tooth technique or the tooth reseeding procedure should, if developed, be able to deal with almost all tooth losses from such accidental happenings.

When we began this section we identified two main ways in which the engineer might be able to extend lifespans. Thus far we have concentrated on methods of stopping or side-stepping deterioration, and not dealt in any depth with the problems of actually identifying sites of mechanical failure.

Although, as we have seen, a great amount of what goes wrong in the body goes wrong in ways which are expected, and can even within limits be predicted, there will undoubtedly be good reasons, even in the harder structures, for finding out exactly how a given system is faring, and whether limits of tolerance to strain are being approached.

The internal monitoring of tissues may seem a very far-fetched idea, but recently in the field of espionage a completely new and revolutionary radio technique has brought the future within touching distance. One great problem in 'bugging' rooms was the amount of current that a radio transmitter, even a minute instrument, needed to keep radiating, and the difficulty of providing a battery small enough to escape detection, and big enough to keep the transmitter on the air. The solution to this may have created a revolution in medical electronics, for a transmitter was designed which had no battery attachment, but drew its power from other powerful stations in the area, transmitting its own data on a different frequency. It was, in effect, a detector and wave-band converter, dependent upon energy it could pick up, and as such it never went off the air except during the periods when the big stations from which it drew its power ceased to transmit.

Such a minute radio transmitter, batteryless and therefore very unlikely to set up reactions in the tissues, or need constant power-pack replacement, could be placed within vital organs, and made to transmit data about the state of its surrounding environment on command. It could be permanently available to give reports, and yet at the same time not inconvenience the life of its wearer. It could be used to prepare reports to be fed into specially designed computers, programmed to compare minute changes in a subject's body over time, and to suggest ways in which these changes could be handled. Such computers might be remote from the wearer, and accept data cabled to them over long distances.

There is no doubt that many of the problems of extended lifespans will be decisional, that is to say, they will have to do with action to be taken at certain stages in accordance with certain prearranged and very complex criteria. Decisional problems always demand facts, and further require the facts to be displayed. In-built, permanent monitoring will provide such facts, and electronic machines the displays.

4

A Self-maintaining Machine

There is a sense in which man already is a good example of a partly self-maintaining machine. Search though we may through the range of man's inventions, we shall not find a material, object, or entity, which so clearly shows this capacity to repair itself, and so stolidly endures the erosion of time.

But there are two reasons why man is not entirely a self-maintaining machine. First, he is a highly complex organism, which is not quite complex enough, and secondly, he is tied to a queer evolutionary programme which does not need him to be immortal to go on functioning.

Making man into a completely self-maintaining machine will not, therefore, be a simple task. On the contrary, it will be the most demanding intellectual and moral struggle that man has ever sought. But the conflict will be won for the excellent reason that the gap that separates man from immortality in the physical sense is finite, but man's capacity for innovation is infinite.

Within the past half century man has made six enormous strides towards immortality. We can list these, and later see in what ways they are likely to influence the developing struggle. They are, in a significant order, advances in his capacity:

1. to examine objects very minutely;
2. to devise a methodology of problem-solving;
3. to simulate, or model, systems or interactions that he cannot see, or would interfere with if he tried to see;
4. to calculate the probable interactions of physiological systems with many different aspects;

5. to monitor and display the results of his studies of minute cellular universes in the body; and
6. to influence very small things with very big forces.

We shall be examining the thrust of these six advances in a later part of this chapter. Meantime, it is only ethical to point out that we have not yet reached the stage of a crusade for ultra-longevity or immortality, launched by motivated biologists. The six thrusts previously mentioned are selected from an overview of research activities which biologists and others are engaged in for relatively limited objectives. Many biologists not only have limited objectives (the extension of the active span of life by ten years, say) they also do not see their own work correlated with that of others. We ought to realize, however, that such piecemeal activities, undertaken often in isolation, with possibly limited aims, or no aims at all, could be the hardware of an immortalist crusade, provided that the funds, the will and the ability to put together research data become available. Indeed we should not expect biologists to be the driving force behind such a crusade. The super-technician, which is what the biologist is, does not have the political skill, the methodological training, or almost by definition the freed vision to push such a movement along. As in the past, this is the task of the politician, or the political technocrat with a quite different range of abilities, and a broader spectrum of contacts. But let us see what is currently known about ageing in a theoretical and practical way.

One of the most significant models for the testing out of ageing theories is somewhat obviously the graph of actual mortality, the curve of survival of a given species over time. If we keep to the date on vertebrates, higher animals with backbones like mammals and reptiles, then we see the same, or nearly the same pattern in all curves. The elapsed span of life is different, of course, because lifespans of different species differ, but the shape of the mortality curve remains much the same. It lifts gradually in early life, demonstrating that a very small number of individuals die at each chosen interval in the youthful period of their lives. But soon it starts to rise in a sharply sloping gradient, and suddenly, or so it would seem, it is shooting up, demonstrating that great numbers of the population are dying at much the same time. Shortly after that it goes off the graph altogether, and the population is completely wiped out.

The overriding implication of this picture is clear enough. It is that the risk of death is cumulative. The longer the life the greater is the risk, until at some stage the probabilities pile up to such an extent that death is unavoidable. We can draw some other conclusions too from this.

One of them is that if dying were controlled by some kind of single clock, and by clock is meant a chemical reservoir in the body that would run dry, then provided this clock ran accurately all members of a species would die on the same day, in the same month, or in the same year, dependent on whether they were flies, mice or men. Some species of very primitive animals do, it seems, have a clock of this kind, and do die all within a day. There is also evidence of clockwork in higher animals, but it is not death clockwork: mammals like man do not die to a calibrated command. They die by an accumulation of defects, which initially is not mortal, but by minimal increases reaches a level of physical incapacity that causes death.

Of course, this conclusion is not the one that the would-be immortalist would choose if he had God at his command and was instructing him in simple and easily repairable design. Death controlled by a clock, or even by a number of clocks, might be much easier to tackle than death as a consequence of accumulation of errors. Man could wind up such a clock or clocks. Now he is faced with the much more difficult task of repairing or preventing a whole universe of small but combining errors. But there is one other point to be made here: if man died at the command of an internal clock we would not expect to find any systems within him that were designed to do repairs. There is, however, evidence of just such a repair system functioning in man. It is not, of course, absolutely efficient, and it is doubtful if it operates continuously, but the fact of its existence is of great significance to the would be immortalist, because it may be a most valuable ally in his struggle to keep alive for ever.

The main thrust of ageing research over the past ten years has been reductionist. That is to say researchers have been trying to break body systems down into smaller and smaller comprehensible processes. Incidentally this research has pressed the limits of conventional biology very hard indeed, in fact, in many cases it has broken clean through into molecular and atomic physics. It is worth noting at this point, because it will become relevant further on, that this reductionist thrust may have to be supplanted by a new interest in holism, in other words by a capacity to understand not only microprocesses but also macroprocesses, the group behaviour of whole systems as opposed to the minute examination of their parts.

It is convenient to deal with the various theories of ageing on a micro to macro basis, in other words to look first at those concerned with the smallest systems of the body, the nuclei of cells, and then to examine, still within the cellular context, those dealing with activities outside the nucleus. Leaving the cell, we can then examine ageing in connective tissues, and finally take a brief look at changes in the very hard structures of the body, the bones and teeth.

There are several things that ought to be said about these ageing theories. First of all we should question their validity, in other words the extent to which they tell us what is really going on in the body. It is highly significant for example that most of the theories conform very well to the mathematical models of survival, constructed from the known ages of a species. But if most of them do this, can they be equally true? How do we pick our way through such strongly competing ideas as these?

The short answer is that they may all be equally true but at different levels of truth. Things that are equal to the same thing are equal to each other, and theories that all satisfy the same criteria are probably very closely related. But how related? One answer could be that they are related in a causal chain, in other words some of the theories may be related to causes and some to effects. This causal chain need not be a simple link-following-link entity. Two theories might explain happenings that were caused by a third factor, itself the subject of a theory. It is this kind of linkage that might enable all the theories to conform to a single criterion, the survival pattern, and still be equally valid.

Once this notion of cause and effect has been introduced, it is also vital to make several other points clear. First there is a sense in which cause is usually seen as having a different and more elevated status than effect. In the field of counter-ageing activities this is not a very helpful distinction. For one thing it may be very difficult to identify any first cause for ageing; the cause/effect chain may be to all intents circular, and it may be necessary to break in upon it, rather than find the end. For another, although we may formally identify one change as cause and another as effect, we may be much more successful in combating effect than in trying to deal with cause. This would not necessarily be a reason for lamentation. On the contrary, if such an effect were appallingly destructive physically, it would be one for congratulation. In sum then we may have to look at identifiable effects a little unconventionally in counter-ageing schemes, because we are after all dealing with the foundation of life itself, on top of which a huge structure of cause-and-effect activity has been built.

First then the cells. There are different kinds of cells in the body, but whatever their function they all have two operational characteristics in common: they have to maintain themselves, if they can, and they have to multiply, if they must. Not all cells do in fact multiply in adult organisms: nerve and muscle cells, for example, a very significant group, do all their multiplying in the foetal stage and none thereafter. This does not mean, of course, that they stay the same size; they are, in fact, engaged in extension and new connection as part of the continuous process throughout their periods of maturation. But in terms of formal relationships one to another they are the same individuals as they were before birth.

Other cells' opportunities for being around for long periods are very limited. Bone marrow cells are being spawned, grown and tossed out at a very fast rate. For them the old adage applies with great severity, 'Before you know where you are, you are somewhere else'.

Between these kind of extremes there are many variations in maintenance ability and rate of multiplication. Some cells, possibly liver cells, multiply and die twice or three times in a human lifetime. From these and from other cells with a similar slow turnover, the body extracts a colossal 'mileage'. The implications of this are quite clear. A cell which has a long 'life', and by 'life' is here meant existence as one identity, has as its main task to keep its internal economy consistent. It has little need to stress itself generating descendants. All it has to do (although this in the end may be impossible) is to keep its internal systems constant. On the other hand a fast turnover cell has two tasks; its own maintenance, and the development of the next generation, with possibly the subordinate role of getting itself off the stage when it has finished its piece without fuss.

Using the very loose terminology of the workshop, cells both keep up their own function and divide to form new cells by a highly sophisticated use of templates. These templates, the working instructions for maintenance and duplication, are inherited as legacies from cell ancestors and, theoretically, provided the templates are exact copies, the functions of cells should not vary from generation to generation. There should be exact replication and precise maintenance.

Templates, in fact, come in two categories. There is the engotype copy, the master design, kept under a cellular lock and key, and brought out to be copied up when the cell is about to divide, so that a similar exact copy for just such a genotype purpose can be passed in to a daughter cell. This genotype copy is a vital element in genetic control. On its unchanging nature depends the continuity and viability not only of the cell, but of the organism to which the cell belongs, and perhaps that of the species to which the organism belongs. It is exceptionally difficult to damage, walled up as it is in its own capsule. But as we shall see, it can be damaged, and when it is damaged the consequences for both cell progeny and organism can be cataclysmic.

Obviously cells that do not divide do not have such a crucial task to defend the integrity of the genotype template. They share, however, with dividing cells the problems of the second category, the working template, and in a sense this is more critical for them. The working templates (there are in fact many copies in each cell) lead an altogether rougher existence. They are the workaday patterns on which the minute-to-minute, hour-to-hour, life of the cell depends. We should not, from a commonsense point of view, expect that designs subject to much wear and tear would remain as precise as the day they were synthesized, and the working templates are no exception to this rule. They do break and vary with the passage of time.

Sited as they are in the industrial areas of the cell, the working templates understandably show change. But there is evidence that the genotype template, even though it is in an ivory tower compared with its working counterpart, also undergoes stresses. In cells with a rapid division rate, of course, the genotype template is in more frequent use anyway, and consequently does not get quite the kid-gloves treatment it receives in the slower dividing environments. But this apart, and even in the cases of cells where the division rate is relatively slow, the genotype template does, it seems, undergo a sort of wear and tear, which although not of the rigour of other genetic components, is significant. One thing is fairly clear, however: genotype template breakdowns do not have the catastrophic effects in ageing terms that they were once thought to have. This does not mean that they are not implicated in certain age-linked diseases like cancer. But as a total explanation of the ageing process they fail, and they fail for two important reasons – firstly that there are probably not enough of them, and secondly that when they do occur they are often strongly selected against, in other words they cause such confusion in cell division, or produce progeny so aberrant that they are eliminated rapidly.

Genotype templates may vary, and working templates may

become ragged with wear. Both then contribute their own inaccuracies to the running mechanisms of the cells, and these inaccuracies can be cumulative in their effects. However, regardless of template accuracy there may be mistakes in the ways in which the instructions are carried out. This is almost the same thing as saying that although the architect's designs were accurate the builders built the house carelessly, but not quite, for with a cell we are not dealing with a once and for all entity like a house which is up and standing, or not standing, as the case may be. A cell has to be continually rebuilt, and in the process of rebuilding there is continual reutilization of parts which may be defective. It is as though the house had to be continually rebuilt under the permanent handicap of a defective lighting system, which eventually created yet another permanent defect, a faulty water system, which in turn, etc., etc., etc.

This is the protein synthesis theory of ageing and it has some evidence to support it. In fact it is a cytoplasmic theory, dealing with happenings within the cell but outside the nucleus, and as such it gives a very useful interpretation of events in an area which we have not as yet covered.

Although some researchers believe that the dynamic processes of ageing start in the cells of the body, we must not neglect other non-cellular structures, and the probable ways in which time eats into their efficiency. In general terms the cells of the body are fixed within various sorts of frames of connective tissue.

Bone cells are, for example, lodged in a frame of collagen and mineral salts that we call bone, but this is one of the rigid structures of the body where there is more framework than cell matter. In other organs such as the liver the reverse situation applies, and the cells dominate.

It is a mistake to think of connective tissue as having a grossly subordinate function, a propping-up status. In fact its tasks are both varied and important. Apart from structure, they include protection, lubrication, shock absorption, storage of water and electrolytes, transport and exchange, maintenance of proper pressures and electrical potentials, all functions that can influence events at a distance, and cause chains of deterioration.

We must however appreciate that cells command connective tissue, even though they subsequently come to depend on it, and that they may be influenced by this tissue and can destroy it, doing so in pursuance of certain programmes of maintenance and repair.

It is probable that much of the ageing of connective tissue is systematic, i.e. that reorderings of molecular structure cause liability to tearing, but at least as much could be the consequence of cell influences. It is important to see therefore that the two phenomena we shall now be discussing in relation to tissue generally, free radicalization and cross linking, may also be deeply implicated in the kinds of changes that we observed in cells. And it is also important to grasp the fact that measures which will be taken to combat them will also affect the operation of cells.

When we burn a piece of paper we set off an irreversible chemical reaction. The molecular structure of the paper alters dramatically, and immediately the burning has finished it reaches a new low free-energy state, from which it will not vary by easily measurable amounts until some new and drastic chemical influence is brought to bear upon it. The paper no longer fulfils the functions of paper, and indeed there is no known way in which it can be made to take up those functions again except indirectly, by an elaborate process of recycling its elements through the tree growth, felling and pulping process. Burning is an excellent method of setting up irreversible chemical changes, and it is probably fortunate that although heat is involved in body processes there is no actual burning, because this would mean that the parts involved in the process would be, in time, irreversibly transformed.

Deterioration processes in the body are however much more akin, in transformation terms, to the weathering and wear of rubber. Rubber loses its long chain molecule spring characteristics as a result of wear and tear, and the disappearance of certain essential chemicals by weathering. But rubber can be reformed into an elastic state by being melted down, chemically treated, and recured. This gives us a clue to the possible ways in which the kinds of quiet wear-and-tear changes that cause connective tissue to change its molecular nature may be tackled in comprehensive anti-ageing programmes. Quiet heating and wearing are energy processes, and the body is a chemical works in which there are a good many processes of chemical exchange, involving energy. The waste products of such processes are various, but one kind, the unstable substances known as free radicals, are particularly damaging.

Free radicalization has very important effects upon tissues. It can start a process of molecular bunching which can be most significant in several sorts of ways. Molecules have an optimum starting pattern in tissue, which has been devised to resist the stresses and strains suffered by the tissue material which they form. In cartilage, for example, the molecular array of the collagen molecules is specifically designed to stop splitting, and if it is patterned in any different way it shows a greater tendency to fray and tear.

In less rigid structures molecular bunching can also lead to build-up of molecular lumps which will not dissolve in the various phases of cell activity, and cannot be broken down. This may cause the accumulation of a coating of a substance akin to varnish on various mechanisms within the cell. Substances such as lipofuscin which may derive from uncontrolled molecular bunching have been observed blocking up heart cells, particularly in nations which have diets that promote free radicalization.

This is perhaps the place to make an important point in relation to the ageing of tissues. Certain organs or parts of organs in the body have been observed to show no signs of ageing over time. That is to say even the minutest microscopic examination demonstrates no difference between specimens taken from old and those taken from young persons. From this and other evidence we can make the following speculative but useful deductions.

Structures in a very low energy state, i.e. those that cannot be oxidized or burnt very easily, are not greatly at risk because their chemical lives are far longer than that of the body. Similarly, structures with a very high free energy state are not at risk either because the fact that their lives are short means that for the body to survive at all they will have to be replaced in a regular schedule. The structures that are important in ageing are those whose lifetimes are the same as that of the body, because they are not short-lived enough to force the body to replace them, and they may on the other hand be fragile enough to contribute to the destruction of the whole system.

We need now to turn to yet another theory, that which holds that the brain and the nervous system are deeply implicated in the ageing process. Statisticians have recently examined longevity and brain size by means of mathematical techniques. They have done this with a variety of mammals of all ages, and although the results cannot be interpreted as a causal certainty there is much in their evidence to show that brain size is a most important determinant of species lifespan – the bigger the brain the longer the life. We can draw several useful deductions from this observation also. The most important is that the brain is deeply involved with body maintenance, that failures in it and its coupled nervous system are multiplied in terms of physical deterioration, and that if its part in the ageing process could be understood in terms of its total function, some very useful rearrangements might be made.

There are probably two very strong factors influencing the brain's maintenance functions. The first of these is the economy of brain functioning which probably only allows a certain number of brain cells to be involved in regulation duties, even though other cells could quite easily do the same job, and may indeed be doing no significant other job at all. The second is the non-dividing nature of nerve cells. A nerve cell does not divide, and therefore lacks the ability to renew itself. It must therefore try to keep itself at a constant function, by means of its own repair systems.

Relatively slight changes in the economy of a nerve cell, changes which do not immediately threaten that cell's existence, may have dynamic effects on other cell systems. Let us take the example of a non-replicating nerve cell, lodged firmly in its connective matrix and part of a highly sensitive conductor linking brain and muscle. As yet we lack full knowledge of the nature of muscle control, particularly in free movements, but what we do know suggests the existence of a complex, electrical pulse, sequence triggering and monitoring movement. Microvoltages are involved and bursts of electrical pulses, which are very easily distorted by arcing, voltage drain and all the other interferences to messages caused by faulty cells.

One of the consequences of the falling off in a nerve cell's efficiency in this kind of situation could be that a muscle ceased to function at full tone, and thus, if this muscle happened to be involved in bone-nutrient circulation, the bone involved would begin to lose density. And one of the consequences of that might be that a hip-bone could break. And so on, and so on. We need not follow the chain any further.

But what we should see is that this is possibly a highly artificial situation and an optimistic one. We ought not to exclude the likelihood that in real life other cellular changes in other systems might, for example, be causing a breakdown in the correction system for poor muscle response, in other words, making the situation much worse.

But now there is one other prominent ageing theory which we must consider, and this claims that ageing is a consequence of errors that the body systems make in identification. The various imperfections in function that creep in, when for example molecules become cross-linked and cells start to fail, are the basis for this theory.

It has become increasingly clear that the body packs a range of self-destructive weapons within its biological armoury. In terms of actual ageing consequences, several actual diseases have been identified which are probably caused by a combination of two processes, a failure to identify cells as part of the body, and a resultant attack upon them. Autoimmune diseases of the aged currently under study include anaemias, diabetes, thyroiditis, and the collagen-type diseases of which rheumatoid arthritis is the most prominent example. In these illnesses the probability is that zealous protection systems are spurred into action by errors that deprive whole organs of their immunity status. The blind battle that follows is the disease. But the point is not so much that mistakes occur at this stage, but that destructive systems exist, because under complete control they might offer a new anti-ageing weapon. If uncontrollable cells threaten the body's viability then it might be possible to deprive them of their immunity status, in order to expose them swiftly to the losing battle that must follow this deprivation.

Research workers already know something of the mechanism of rejection, the phenomenon in which the body recognizes and destroys alien tissue introduced into it, usually in the shape of grafts, transplants, or most often bacteria. The mechanism seems to involve the activity of the lymphocyte, the lymph tissue cell, which usually has duties connected with tissue drainage and circulation; at least the simple view of the rejection phenomenon implicates the lymphocyte, and suggests that it is triggered to invade and destroy grafted tissue by fragments of material that drop off the graft itself. Certain more recent experiments have however indicated that rejection may not be an assigned task, which the lymphocytes are sent off to perform, but that all cells are capable of rejection activity when they meet up with alien organisms, the rejection being caused by some kind of micro-molecular friction – incompatible cells rubbing against each other.

This is now the point to discuss various ways in which an integrated repair and correction system can be built to ensure that the body does not deteriorate. In any such design the intention would be to make maximum (and by maximum is meant beyond normal limits) use of the body's own systems of repair.

To begin, in general terms, it is clear that the body does a considerable amount of obvious repair. What is not so obvious is the work it does in systems that are hidden from view, or where the consequences are not clear. And what is not obvious at all is the range of repair it would achieve if it were pressed.

Let us take the cell first. Template repair or protection should be broadly divisible into two fields, the problems of the master template (the genotype) and those of the working templates (metabolic D.N.A.). Unfortunately, though we make this division in a formal sense it is difficult to separate evidence for repair or damage into separate compartments, and we shall have to content ourselves with evidence which may involve both kinds of template.

One vital element in template stability is environmental balance. In plants, for example, light intensity, temperature, the moisture content of the soil and the electrolite balance of the nutrients in the plant's food are all vital factors. Next, genetic research has shown that in some, but not necessarily all living systems there are mutator genes actually in the master template system. The exact nature of the action of these genes is not known, but they may make a chemical which affects the master template. Thirdly there is the effect of radiation, which can be seen in two contexts. There is the problem of natural radiation both from the earth and from the universe, which is in amount very small, but which affects every living creature and has hitherto been largely overlooked. Artificial radiation, specifically that generated by X-ray machines and accelerators, is known to damage templates. A huge range of experiments has been carried out, where radiation was used to damage templates with a view to discovering how fast and how far the organism can repair the damage. Most of these begin with a relatively young subject, usually a small mammal such as a rat, irradiate it, and then assess the rate with which the damaged templates are repaired.

Usually the results show that template damage can be repaired, provided there is not too much of it too quickly administered. But a much more significant set of experiments has been carried out with organisms – on human liver cells that have aged naturally. Using a different and very poisonous hydrocarbon compound it was possible to revitalize the livers of these patients, indicating that in some way not clearly understood the liver cell templates which had become defective, and would not naturally have repaired themselves, became sufficiently stimulated by the poison to do under pressure what they would not do under their own volition.

If there are such things as mutator genes, or if some of the other genetic material in the cell is found to be the trigger for an ageing process, we may be able to tackle the template malfunction in another very promising way. We may be able to use viruses which have a special effect upon the wayward or malignant gene. Already it is known that the Shope virus has a very specific effect upon the cells of the liver, causing them to make more than a normal amount of aginase, an enzyme vitally important in brain development. This introduced the idea of using the Shope virus as a kind of surgical probe to ginger up the gene or genes in the liver which are responsible for the sort of mental deficiency that a lack of aginase produces. Viruses and genes are much of a size, at least in terms relative to the infinitesimal world in which they operate. Viruses can gain entry to cells with great ease (they have a special design which facilitates this) and they are selective, entering some kinds of cells, but not others. It is quite possible that we may be able to alter viruses so that they will become even more selective and thus pick and choose between cells.

Primitive but successful attempts have also already been made to extend the life of cells under highly artificial conditions. In one case red blood cells, taken for transfusion, were found to lose an essential enzyme in storage, and to deteriorate at a rate linked with the loss. Added to the cell suspension the synthetic enzyme inosine had a dramatic effect on the red cells. Their life-span trebled, and then they succumbed to the effects of other losses or transformations that inosine did not prevent.

Another attempt was even more artificial, but even more interesting in its scope and results. It has long been known that the cellular effects of exposure to X-rays closely mimics that of actual ageing, though it is not an exact equivalent. An opportunity therefore exists to test out ways in which the effects of X-ray radiation can be minimized and, in an approximate sense, those of natural ageing also. Research in this case showed that feeding mice with radioprotective substances did protect them against the acute effects of radiation. But there was another consequence of this experiment, in its essence less reassuring. Although the acute effects were diminished, the long-term effects were just as severe. Some cell systems had therefore obviously not been protected.

We can also make another prediction, one which generally relates to all life-prolonging activities, and one which can be made with some confidence, because it is based upon facts that can be clearly observed in various experiments. This is that if there is one overriding deduction to be made about attempts to stabilize cellular activities, it is that balance is vital.

Life prolongation is an attempt at a steady state for a large number of different systems very sensitive to normal environmental variations, and probably all too prone to start up, or fail to stop, ageing processes, if the environment varies too much.

Natural living is a very steady process, in which there is a constant, but in the end unsuccessful struggle to strike and hold balances. Unnatural living seems to intensify both the risk and the struggle. Researchers have noticed that cells grown outside the body for immortality in culture media are fantastically sensitive to light, heat and changes in the nutrients with which they are fed. It has also been discussed that relatively small temperature alterations, which cause rats to live at a new and less demanding metabolic rate, can hold up the processes of ageing and cellular disease. What this means is that any anti-ageing machine must have regard for cell environments, the status and efficiency of connective tissue in which cells are set, and the limits within which they can work efficiently.

There is some evidence, but it is by no means confirmed, that the more specialized cells of the body have powers of repair far in excess of their less specialized brethren. This is partly connected with the fact that a characteristic of some non-specialized cells such as those forming bone marrow is their tremendous speed of reproduction. This makes it possible for repair to become a very insignificant feature of cell life, since before a cell has a chance to become defective it is replaced. But of course this is not necessarily the case with a specialized cell, which if it is a neurone (a nerve cell), for example, may have no replacement on hand.

The design for any artificial cell repair system may therefore have to include equipment to gain an accurate knowledge of two situations.

a. Whether in the case of cells which have no repair facilities, reproduction is keeping pace with deterioration;
b. How far cells which can repair themselves are, in fact, managing to keep up their efficiency over time.

There is probably no more significant area for examination than the body's nervous system. We must in fact look at this inability of nerve cells to divide in several different ways. First off, there seems to be little doubt this inability is highly important in ageing because it places on a vital system the burden of an impossibly high level of self-maintenance, a burden which cannot be sustained, and the non-sustaining of which has consequences for other dependent systems some of which ironically enough may not have to keep up the same standards, because they can divide.

As to the reasons for non-division of nerve cells there is an interesting range of hypotheses. Non-dividing cells may lack dividing capability because their function is too complex for replication; certainly this seems to be a rational view of the status of brain cells, which may carry a mass of learned material, very difficult to replicate. Whether it applies to other nerve cells in other parts of the body is another matter, but if it should be shown that all nerve cells have to follow a brain-cell fashion, for matters of biological convenience rather than necessity, then this would be a most profound discovery. It might open the door to a whole new strategy of intervention.

The involvement of the nervous system in the process of ageing is both causal and amplifying. This means that changes in its cells and probably in its cell-to-cell connections have severe effects on the integrity of organs under their control. Even in cases where nerve-cell deterioration is not a primary cause, occurring as it does in feedback and monitoring circuits, it will intensify organ deterioration and probably make local attempts at repair more difficult.

All successful immortality machines will therefore have to give the nervous system first priority. For this they will have a wide range of sophisticated electronic testing devices including an instrument which will simultaneously test the electrical sensitivity of groups of nerves, comparing their performances with standards, and displaying the results of these tests together with facts about the rate, and site, of deterioration. This instrument will be capable of artificial stimulation, in other words it will be able to arrange for tests to be run on nerve circuits, possibly not in common use, whose effectiveness may well be slowly dropping off. It will, of course, be an external instrument, involving the minimum of probes, and depending on an advanced technique of selective induction, using electromagnetic methods of putting power into nerves in the body, rather in the way that a transformer passes power from coil to separated coil.

In creating this first stage of the immortality machine man may discover that the body's knowledge of what repairs are needed, and its capacity to answer these needs, are in step – and it acts only on what it knows. Then there may be the opposite of this situation in which the body's repair capacity far exceeds its knowledge of what to do. This is a possibility though not a likely one, but if it should prove to be so then it would open up a considerable range of induced repairs, provided always of course that ways could be found to direct the unused repair potential. Finally there is a chance that the body knows of more needs than it can satisfy. This last has the merits of being the most logical in developmental terms, in that evaluation seems to precede action in most human activities, and, of course, it opens up the possibility that artificial repair may be directed by the intimately involved monitoring system of the body.

At present we know very little indeed about the range of monitoring that the brain carries out. But there is a distinct possibility that a vast amount of monitoring goes on though the results may not be easily accessible. As has been suggested earlier, the brain may only concern itself with matters it can do something about, but this need not prevent it incidentally getting hold of much superfluous information. In every piece of information there is, after all, a great amount of formal redundancy, dependent to some extent on the use that is being made of it. If we can devise equipment to listen in to all the internal traffic, much in the same way that an electronic eavesdrop is organized for espionage, then we may be able to rework the facts we glean in the light of facts we derive from other sources. This is a kind of body espionage which bears some resemblance to real espionage in that it depends upon the inter-relationship of items of information that may have very little value in themselves, and indeed little value to their authorized recipient, but when taken in conjunction with other facts suddenly reveal or confirm a blinding new theory.

Monitoring is the single task of presenting or displaying information. But it forms part of a much wider brief for decision taking, in fact there is a sense in which it is a dominant factor in decision making.

Monitoring in effect must not only detect the malfunctions of cellular systems, it has also to compare the data that it gleans with a mass of other information, which relates not only to the body under examination but also to the theory and modelling of the ageing process. In particular it needs to be able to decide whether a given ageing system:

a. will correct or repair itself, or stabilize unrepaired at a new level;
b. will deteriorate further and affect other systems, or collapse quietly and insignificantly.

Strategies for correction may also require an accurate knowledge of priority needs. Systems may only be tackleable in a sequence, and thus it is possible that monitoring may also have to determine the time-scale of any deterioration/reparation process, so that the most effective strategy can be planned. It may also involve a substantial amount of cell or organ simulation.

Cell simulation is a jargon phrase which covers an enormously wide potential field. In essence it means the technique of reproducing all the elements of cellular activity in mathematical terms, boiling down the exchanges, conversions, and syntheses of the cell's economy to the code of mathematics. Once this can be done, and it has already been done for less complicated 'machines', a new and vital tool is available to fight mortality. Once a machine, albeit a machine of quietly moving fluids and solutions, has been brought down to equational form, it can be 'run' in a computerized form. Within the computer, of course, the cell becomes a set of transistors and circuits triggered by a programme, but it is soon working its own programme, an electrical entity mimicking its real counterpart. And then, of course, it should be possible to simulate not only the working of a single cell but also the interaction of cells with each other.

Let us assume then that not only with nerve cells, but also in other types, we can perfect techniques to force a recopy or renewal of templates, and that at the same time we can ensure that the fair copy will remain absolutely intact. Unfortunately we cannot assume permanent perfection in cell working from such a system; indeed, commonsense if nothing else would suggest that there must be by-products of normal cell chemistry whose existence and effects must be significant in the ageing process.

We know from the earlier discussion that unstable molecular fragments known as free radicals occur in and around cells. A free radical is a chemical unit that contains an unpaired electron, and the result of having such an electron unpaired is that the unit becomes unusually prone to set off oxidizing and cross-linking reactions, reactions which probably have an extremely damaging effect on the cell's structure.

Fortunately we already possess two most important pieces of knowledge which may enable us to deal with the problem. To begin with we have a technique of measuring how much free radicalization is taking place in and around cells. An unpaired electron does not orbit a true path round its nucleus; it flips about like a spacecraft out of control, and as it does its flipping, it gives out a characteristic noise or resonance which can be picked up by very delicate detectors. Electron spin resonance measurement is a powerful tool for detecting abnormalities at the molecular level in cells and tissues.

However there are serious problems involved in using it to screen whole organs which may be made up of millions of cells. To begin with there is the difficulty of obtaining the sample, and retaining it in such a way as to shield it from the interference of other cells. Hitherto E.S.R. measurements have been made '*in vitro*', that is to say on cell samples maintained outside the body, where it is relatively easy to control the situation and stop interference. It may be necessary to overcome at least three major problems before E.S.R. can be a useful tool in monitoring cell and tissue ageing.

1. The problem of data interpretation. Different resonance patterns may have to be coded to different elements in the cell, and patterns of correct working and malfunction recognized.
2. The problem of '*in vivo*' (in the living body) sampling. This may invoke a most elaborate electromagnetic shielding technique.
3. The statistical problem of sampling, i.e. what percentage of an organ, cells and tissues, must be sampled to give an accurate prediction of the ageing state of that organ.

The second step would then be to neutralize, or eliminate, these free radicals before they set off damaging reactions. There might be various approaches to this. We do, in fact, know quite a lot about the unmonitored control of free radicalization, because for some years there has been a need to preserve stocks of foods made with fats and oils. Free radicals, which speed up deterioration in these products, have been identified and scavenged for by means of highly complex new chemicals of the toluene family. One of these, B.T.H. (butylated-hydroxytoluene) was found to be such a powerful scavenger, and so dramatic in its effect upon free-radicalized tissues in living things, that it doubled the life span of mice.

Tissues that are oxidized or develop cross-linkage are changed of course. Perhaps they are not changed quite so drastically as burned paper or rusted iron, but they may at least be as altered as perished rubber. We can see how irreversibly altered is burnt paper with no possibility, save by an elaborate recycling process, of retrieving its paper-like characteristics. Oxidized iron (rust) can be reconverted to iron by heating with hydrogen; perished rubber can be reconstituted by being cooked with an alkali. But these drastic processes would be of no use in the body. Might there then be gentler ways of reversing age-linked changes in body tissues?

Enzymes are extremely powerful agents for change, any small quantities of which can have extremely drastic results. They are produced in the body, in plants and artificially. Recently a very powerful enzyme named Beta-amizopropionitrile (B.A.P.N.) has been discovered, one of the properties of which is an ability to split up a molecular cross-linkage. B.A.P.N. has, in fact, remarkable effects on lengthening the lifespans of mice whose diet has been adjusted to give the maximum opportunity for cross-linkage to build up within them.

Enzymes are, in fact, quite extraordinary substances. Briefly they cause body chemical reactions to take place, at temperatures and under conditions which would need most elaborate and difficult experiments to arrange artificially. They seem to work by an incredibly precise system of molecular bonding, similar in analogy to a frictionless gear chain requiring little energy to set and keep in motion.

It might be possible to develop all kinds of new enzymes by a process of selective cultivation. In essence this would involve sampling different sorts of cross-linked material, and allowing it to be used as a food by any one of a range of micro-organisms for whom it would be the only source of nourishment. This would force enzymes in the micro-organisms to show their reproductive paces or die, and a very sharp competitive situation would develop, which might lead to strong enzyme strains surviving. But if our counter-ageing programmes are going to make use of the present and future range of powerful chemicals, whether of the catalytic enzyme or the compound-seeking nitrite form, we shall probably need to know a great deal more about methods of actually bringing the chemical to the appropriate site of deterioration.

At the moment our methods are probably very crude. We can feed and inject these chemicals. We can also arrange for the non-enzymes to be breathed in a gaseous form. But we do not know the actual transport methods whereby the chemicals reach the sites. In particular, we do not know if organ interventions or counter activities or inefficiencies will reduce the effect of the chemicals. All these things we shall have to know, and very accurately too.

Fortunately we are beginning to develop tracer techniques with greater and greater refinement. These depend upon the discovery that chemicals made radioactive can be tracked in the body, and followed through all sorts of processes without losing their label. Anti-ageing techniques will also probably include a very sophisticated development of high-pressure gas induction for treating tissue deterioration. It is already known, for example, that it is possible for human beings to breathe unusual gases if they are in a high-pressure environment, and it is also known that very fundamental changes in the gas balance of the blood, and other systems, can be induced by alterations in environmental pressure. It is possible that the efficiency of some of the complicated anti-oxidization, radical scavenging chemicals like B.T.H. may be vastly increased if they can be administered in gaseous form, that is if their complicated chemical structure can resist transformation into gas. But already some very complicated gases have been developed in the chemical warfare field, gases which seem to hold their structure adequately, and which are extraordinarily potent in their effect upon the human body. We can also envisage the possibility that these gases will be isotoped, in other words that they will be made relatively radioactive, which will give a continuous check on their efficiency.

Enzyme therapy on the other hand might be organized into three phases. First the body temperature could be brought down so that the enzyme might be introduced in an inactive state. Then the body temperature could be lifted so that the enzymes went into action, and began to break down cross-linked substances in tissue. Then the body temperature could be lifted to normal levels which would kill off all the enzymes and thus stop the process before it went too far and started destroying vital structure. Of course, the enzymes might have to be assisted in penetration of cell structure if there was too much cross-linked substance for them to dissolve, and in these difficult cases they might be lubricated in by a specially synthesized 'carrier chemical'.

Let us now examine the two-stage design for a self-maintaining machine, as is seen in Figures 6 and 7. Of course this is not a machine in the sense of a nuts and bolts or moving-parts device, although such mechanisms are bound to develop from ideas of this kind. It is a design or a demonstration of a possible method of tackling immortality in which there is a sequence of processes, each screening four different aspects of ageing.

If we examine the first stage which deals with the age stabilization of the central nervous system, a strategy becomes clear. This is to eliminate ageing in the central nervous system, by a multi-screening sequence, to stimulate it to repair other body systems, and to tap its stores of information to help anti-ageing treatments at later stages.

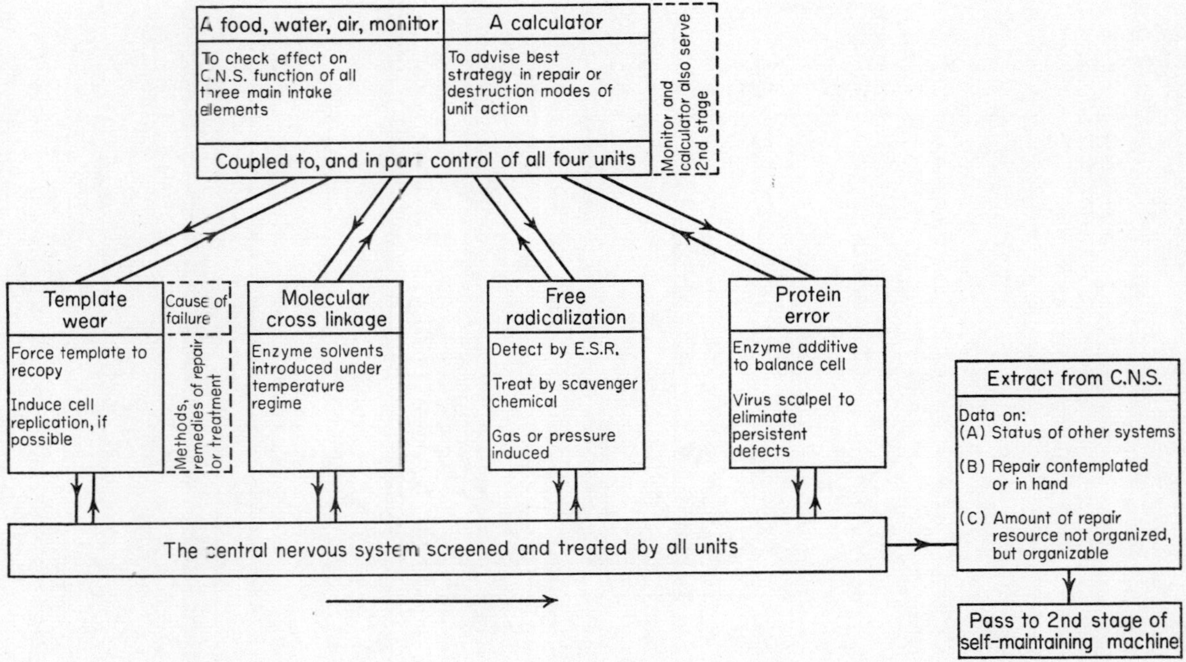

Fig. 6

Preliminary Screen for the Central Nervous System

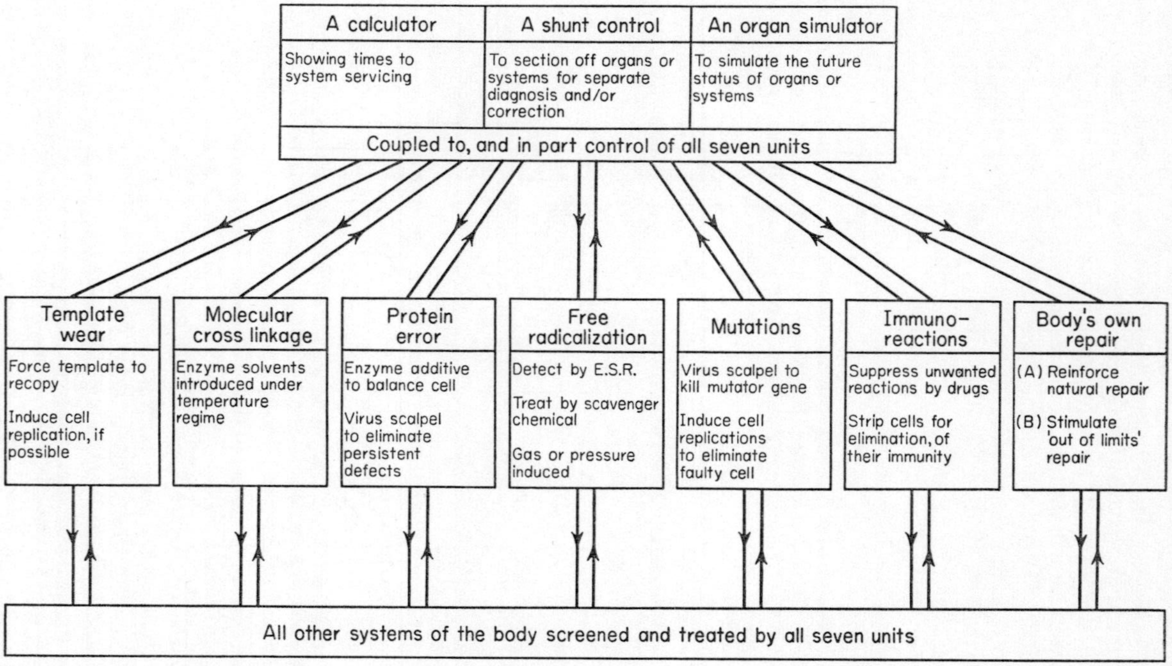

Fig. 7

Secondary Screen for Remaining Body Systems

Overriding the four screening units we see an intake monitor and a calculator. The intake monitor checks the effect on the central nervous system function of three main intake elements, air, food and water. It will also check other minute intakes such as radiation. It will do this by means of minute probes within the body which all transmit data to its analyser. The intake monitor will also receive information from the four screening units, and provide them with data.

The calculator, to which the intake monitor is coupled, will provide a somewhat different service. It will assimilate information from a great range of screens, and work at strategies. For example, it may be able to simulate, and then advise on the possible consequences of destroying a nerve cell and the chances of its regeneration. It will probably be able to present a choice of strategies and show a range of possibilities for every choice.

Second in the hierarchy comes the screening units, four in number at this stage, screening and treating within their own field of ageing process. Their suggested activities are noted in the boxes within the divisions 'cause of failure' and 'methods and remedies'. The units appear to be working simultaneously and co-operatively, but this is a speculation. They may interfere with each other, undo each other's work, unless precautions are taken, or be sequentially dependent. This is the reason why they are connected to the calculator.

The central nervous system is thus screened and treated. How long this process would take is uncertain. It is probable that it would involve regular screening visits to a centre, where information already held on the status of the body could be compared with that obtained from the in-body probes. Certainly this first stage would be expected to provide much information on the status of bodily systems outside the central nervous system which could be passed to the second stage of a self-maintaining machine.

If we now examine the second stage of the machine, it is clear that much the same design has been followed, but with certain elaborations or additions. Once again the calculator and the organ simulator figure boldly at the head of the design hierarchy, joined at this stage by a shunt control to section off organs or systems for separate diagnosis or correction. There is an implication here that the kind of screening/treatments necessary at this second stage will be of a more radical and prolonged kind than previously. Aspects of organ deterioration that a continuously rejuvenated central nervous system cannot prevent are likely to require radical treatment. The areas and volumes of tissue involved will also be much larger.

Three new screening boxes have been added, those of Mutations, Immuno-reactions and Body's Own Repair. Of these, the first two screen either specially applicable organs or organs outside the central nervous system which perform a great deal of cell replication. Body's own repair is in a kind of limbo, but is an important one, between the first and second stages, because it is still very unclear what commands such repair systems, and it may well be that the central nervous system also has its own inbuilt repair programme.

However, the underlying purpose of the inclusion is clear enough. It is to show the necessity for pressing the repair possibilities to their utmost, and if necessary beyond. Pressing beyond may involve damage to other organs, or possibly running down of vital nutrients. But provided the calculators at both stages are functioning correctly, and give accurate advice, it may be possible to boost from external sources depleted stocks or to shut down, temporarily, other organ functions, and carry these artificially.

Both stages 1 and 2 are very closely coupled. Again, though they may seem to be a sequence, central nervous system first, and other organs second, we must not assume that this is mandatory. On the contrary, in some cases it may be necessary to begin at the end and look back to the beginning. In fact this flexibility in method and process will have to be a guideline for all self-maintaining machine designs.

5

Telescoped Brains

The sustaining theme of this study so far has been the prospect that, in the not-too-distant future, man will be able to choose between living a normal lifespan or having the process of his mental and physical ageing halted. At this point in time it would be unwise to assume that absolute immortality would necessarily result from the development of such a halting or suspension technique. The period of halt might be a century, five centuries, or much more, but even while this fantastic period of time elapsed the processes of ageing might move forward in infinitesimally small steps, indetectable by normal means, or at least means that allowed a normal life.

The possibility that ostensible immortality might by tiny defects become mortality again prompts speculation about the prospects of a different kind of immortality, one which could be derived from brain-to-brain transfers. The theory behind such speculation is quite simple.

As the processes of ageing progress in an older person (the theory is not incompatible with the notion of very slow ageing) so preparations are made to transfer his thoughts to another younger brain. In fact, the theory also presupposes some selectivity to the process, and total transfer would seem to be out of the question.

It also presupposes further transfers, and a state of multiple mind, since, as time elapses, more and more bodies will fail, and parts of more and more minds will have to be transferred. But the overriding supposition, and as we shall see the most questionable, is that by selective mental transfer, identity itself could be preserved.

At this point we have to do a little preliminary clearing of the ground and look at the way in which terms are used, anticipating the possible scientific tangles into which too loose a phrasing may lead us.

When the would-be immortalist says, 'I would like to preserve my identity indefinitely' what, in fact, he may be saying is, 'I should like continuously to have experiences which relate to my specific history, location, and position in time'. He is not to be blamed for using the word 'identity' in this way. In fact, he is performing conventionally. Terms like 'identity', 'consciousness', 'intelligence', 'will', 'feeling', are all convenient shorthand for the economical handling of observed behaviour. To describe them thus is not to denigrate them, for without them, and some agreement as to the way in which they could be used, communication would become an interminable set of descriptions.

To take an example: for 'when I regained consciousness after my accident' the equivalent would be a rigmarole of reminiscences about how 'I felt the pain of my bruised head, heard the sound of the ambulance man's voice', etc., etc.

But the trouble with terms like 'identity' is that they take more upon themselves than they can justify by works, and they are used in a kind of magical way, as if they had a kind of privileged life of their own, distinct from the behaviour they are meant to describe. In particular, they tend to be restricted – a man chasing a woman is displaying an effort of will, but a guided missile chasing a plane is not.

By the end of this discussion we shall see that some of these distortions have a particularly confusing effect, making it difficult to grasp or accept concepts that the terms ought to cover but do not, and setting up distinctions that do not stand up to scrutiny. But let us begin by examining the brain mechanisms which create and link the behavioural experiences that we have to describe in such blanket but satisfying terms.

It is almost certain that all our thinking, feeling, imagining, deciding, seeing – the whole range of activities that seem to be both external and internal, in the sense that sounds, etc., seem to come to us from without while impulses are from within – are perceived in electrical impulses and resonances occurring within the brain. A smell is a set of immediate impulses, a well-remembered smell is a retrieval of an old set of impulses, and a smell does not exist, as far as we are concerned, without its impulses, for we have no experience of it without them. It is almost impossible for even the most sophisticated of minds to grasp the significance of this, because all of us are possessed of the quiet delusion (itself a set of impulses) that mental activity is something more, and *needs* to be something more than impulses. But, in fact, we should be glad that this is a delusion, because the existence of precisely translateable sense data means that we can store experience within manageable circuitry and, provided we can reactivate the circuits, have the experience for as long as memory lasts.

How do we begin the process of converting external and internal experience into impulses? In the beginning the baby is bombarded with stimuli, but in the beginning also the baby is equipped with mechanisms to convert those stimuli into coded pulses of electrical energy, which have to be organized, interpreted and stored. The baby is initially equipped with certain rudimentary brain mechanisms which we can call job assemblies; very primitive, but capable of enormous elaboration, capable of interpreting at least enough of the incoming pulses to keep the baby in close touch with the environment.

For example, the pulse code pattern which is the mother's voice is rapidly decoded as a favourable stimulus, perhaps compared with other stimuli, models of which have been inherited, and possibly used as a trigger to set off responses in the baby, such as smiling or gurgling.

This is an example of a very primitive, early-developing job assembly, but in fact the concept is useful to describe other later much more elaborate systems. For example, there is a job assembly for speech recognition which picks up incoming auditory pulses and compares them with bits of word sounds previously heard. As more and more pulses come in, so the probability of a sensible match increases, and finally as a result of a process of weighing probabilities, the job assembly picks an appropriate word. The word (or it can be a phrase) exists as an electrical potential in a microcircuit, and the job assembly activates it by making it resonate. As it resonates so it is heard.

This process is obviously taken through at a colossal speed, and the actual matching is probably done on a basis of the least number of pulse cues needed to set the right word resonating. It is a kind of instantaneous or near-instantaneous search technique, by which a relatively large number of likely matches to the beginnings of pulse cue and word are whittled down to a single correct selection, when later parts are received.

Job assemblies are the workaday organizations of the brain.

They are very rigid structures, mostly not under conscious control, and closely linked with the physical systems of the body. In the strict sense, the amount they contribute to the feeling of conscious identity is obscure. Probably they provide a sense of psychic boundary, and not much more. But the brain holds more intricate and individualized mechanisms, and the most elaborate and specialized of all these we can term the recall assemblies.

Recall assemblies retain our personal history. They have many of the characteristics of job assemblies, being probably organized on the same basis of search probabilities and near-instantaneous matchings. And they have actual elements in common. For example, we may assume that some of the matching syllable-sound fragments that are used to 'hear' a given word, from any source, have as their original models the voice of mother, since mother's voice is the first a child listens to with any degree of attention. Mother's voice therefore exists both as an element in the job assembly for auditory patterns, and in the mother recall assembly.

Recall assemblies, however, have certain characteristics of their own which should be emphasized. First, it is probable that they are largely self-sequence, controlled, that is, so that instead of being heavily dependent upon external stimuli or internal physiological stimuli for their triggering like the job assemblies, their sequence is associational, each recall assembly activating another according to a kind of electrical logic. Then they are probably a good deal more dynamic than job assemblies, having the continuous ability to pick, influence, or exclude elements in other assemblies. And lastly, but probably most important, it is they that have the onus of maintaining identity.

The job assembly performs a vital semi-automatic function, and may well 'command' at times the activities of a recall assembly. But it is likely that in its action, and, what is more important, in the sensation of its activity, there is no difference between individuals. One person (allowing for amplitude) probably hears much the same as another in terms of the activities of their respective job assemblies. But the experiences which differentiate them as individuals come from the content of their respective recall assemblies as a result of what they hear or see being compared and contrasted with what they as individuals have seen or heard in the past.

We can gain some idea of the possible workings of the system if we consider the nature of a given recall assembly that we can call 'Mother'. Obviously in most people this is a huge organization consisting of all sorts of different memories laid down at various developmental stages, such as the warmth of mother, the voice of mother, the various specific and non-specific visual circuitory patterns which enable mother to be recognized visually, plus the admonitions and characteristics of mother; and much else besides that we call to mind at will. And then there is possibly an equally large, disassociated section of the Mother-recall assembly that we cannot bring back to mind, but which is connected with Mother, possibly in a paradoxical way, or in a way which does not harmonize with the dominant assembly feeling about her – the unconscious, or unacceptable things that have become disconnected at some time and for some reason, and are not retrievable by usual means.

The actual electrical ways in which recall assemblies, large and small, operate are still very obscure. Obviously there is a system for 'broad call', when a whole cluster of events or facts is required, and a 'narrow call', when the amount of material is small. The mnemonic situation, when a man remembers his mother in a great auditory, tactual and visual sweep, by comparison with that when he tries to recapture the Christian name of her cousin, are excellent examples of these.

We also have to distinguish two other dimensions of recall, the 'directed', when deliberate attempts are made to move from one concept to another in the situation, say, of an examination, when theories and facts have to be written down in a logical sequence, and the 'free', when memories come flooding back without a conscious directional effort.

Directed thought is probably the observer's, i.e. the thinker's, view of the workings of his recall assembly when that assembly is being held in the foreground of consciousness for long periods. The apparent logical direction of thinking (one thing leading to another) could be a chronological feature; in other words, in addition to the assembly pulse code each item may be individually tagged with a pulse code that relates to the time at which the item was first perceived. Items close in time may be close in pulse-code relationship, and not therefore very likely to set up inter-resonances because of minute irregularities of pulse.

Undirected thought, on the other hand, may depend on items continuing to resonate for minute time spans after the general pulse of a given assembly has tailed away. Although the assembly identifying pulse may be unique to an assembly, the rest of the identifying pulse data may not, and more than one assembly may use it. It could happen therefore that items continuing to resonate beyond a general assembly time are set off by some mechanism items which, although not absolutely identical to them in other assemblies, yet have enough resemblance to be triggered.

It seems to be a logical speculation that if anything is to be transferred from brain to brain it will have to be wholes or parts of recall assemblies. Job assemblies, which are at best the automatic or semi-automatic mechanisms keeping the brain linked with the external world, would of course be available in the brain of the recipient.

It is therefore proposed that the design for a machine to perform the brain transfer will approximate to diagram A, that it will be divided into two main sections. The first will consist of a mapping unit to survey the circuitry of the donor's brain, an extractor to gather circuitry data, and an assembly simulator to hold that data. This section will be linked to a second, with its own mapping unit to survey the recipient's brain, an assembly simulator connected to the first unit to hold the transfer, and finally an inputer to feed the data in.

At this point we have to answer the objection that with sophisticated electronic equipment there would be no necessity to imagine a machine that acted as a kind of intermediary between brain and brain, and that the most likely method would be a direct one, with assemblies being transferred from brain to brain without any organization or storage.

This objection ignores certain difficulties that are almost certain to be met. The first, but not necessarily the most important, is the assumption that assembly matching, donor to recipient, will be a swift process like a blood transfusion. In fact this is a poor analogy, because with blood the transfusion process is dealing with a relatively unchanging substance, unlike an assembly, which is a wave of electrical resonances.

Assembly transfer may be very time-consuming, with much mapping of circuit areas necessary before transfer takes place, and such mapping may be more conveniently done within a machine. Then, of course, a donor may die before his assemblies can be matched up with those of a recipient, and his only chance of immortality will therefore depend upon an intermediate machine holding assemblies, so to speak, until a recipient can be found and mapped.

Mapping micro-circuits within a given assembly (assuming that one assembly only will be taken for implant) may well be a very time-consuming process. For circuits to be identified for implant they will need to be obvious, and this will mean that the chosen assembly will have to be 'in thought' as much as possible.

Diagram A

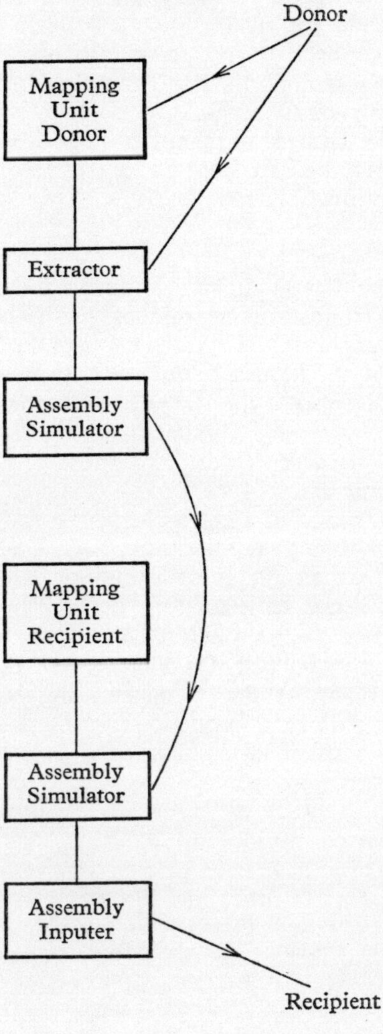
Donor
Mapping Unit Donor
Extractor
Assembly Simulator
Mapping Unit Recipient
Assembly Simulator
Assembly Inputer
Recipient

This would necessitate the creation of a sort of artificial obsession, since in normal persons there is undoubtedly a mechanism that keeps assemblies from reforming, and will even block off continuous stimuli designed to bring the same assembly back to consciousness again and again. Such a defence mechanism will have to be disconnected, and remain in abeyance, while the selected assembly is continuously providing information about its constituent circuitry.

The actual mechanisms of mapping must of necessity be very speculative. It may be that giant electronic models of the donor and recipient brain will have to be built, using billions of microcircuits.

What will this super-computer be like? The first misconception of it could well be that its circuitry will have the same constraints within electrical engineering techniques that limit the capabilities of our present machines. The assembly simulator, for example, may have to copy the human brain, not only in terms of outputs and sequences but also in the very materials that make it up. In other words, the assembly simulators may need to be built of carbon not silicon compounds, and their conductors will be liquids and not metals.

A whole new range of electro-chemistry skills may need to be developed for this, to say nothing of the necessity of solving the more elaborate problems of computer climate. Then the current idea of series construction, the practice of sequential processing of data, will probably have to be discarded. The human brain is probably full of millions of tiny radio transmitters partially independent of central control and capable of transmitting on very different frequencies, perhaps simultaneously. This presupposes the construction of a grossly parallel kind of computer with a tremendous amount of electro-magnetic activity occurring on many different wave bands. Cyberneticists have called this a pandemonium design, though at the moment the only models they have been able to construct of it have been related to job assembly functions. For example, they have been able to recreate the act of seeing an object, where the visual stimulus pattern of that object has to be compared with various existing internal models. Job assembly efficiency puts a high premium on beating the system – in other words, being able to anticipate what the object is before all the data to identify it comes in. Inspired guessing in fact is the mode.

Cyberneticists have been able to envisage a situation in which a kind of controlled pandemonium takes place, namely a yell of different guesses as to what has come in, and what is to come in, from a myriad microcircuit throats. The loudest and longest yell in this situation wins the day, and action is taken on its guess as to what the object is.

The super-computer will also probably be very large, and will need a grand assortment of other machines to tell it about itself, in particular to inform it about its environment and tasks – how, for example, the mapping of the donor is proceeding, what the power requirements are likely to be for completing the assignment, and a myriad of other monitoring essentials.

Now it has been argued that transfer of recall assemblies would by definition be impossible because an assembly in transfer would lose consciousness, and be incapable of resuscitation when the transfer was complete. This view assumes that 'consciousness' is some kind of permanent quality in a circuit, which cannot be passed on, or transferred.

There is, of course, as we have seen, more than one way of talking about 'consciousness' as a phenomenon. We can view it strictly operationally; in other words, we can ask the man in a motor accident who says, 'I recovered consciousness' to say what he actually felt, and we can see when he relates his initial post-accident experiences (hearing the ambulance man's voice, etc.) that what he means by 'consciousness' is the sequence of his waking sensations, whether these be in terms of voices or discomforts.

We can also look at it as a connection phenomenon. Connection-phenomenon theorists hold that the entity that connects experiences, or assembly changes, is a kind of transitional electrochemical state between thoughts, when a brain is neither one thing nor another but something in between. Connection theorists therefore identify 'consciousness' as the transition phase between assembly changes.

None of these theories seem necessarily to exclude the possibility that transfers will be possible. From a purely operational standpoint the recipient of the assembly will have his 'consciousness' altered slightly in quality but not at all in quantity, by being able to fantasize or recall someone else's experience. From a connection standpoint the transplanted assembly will blend with the recipient's mind ready to provide its own quota of transitional 'consciousness' when it goes in and out of thought.

In the case of the permanent-quality theorists it is possible that they are talking about a sort of 'consciousness' that is in a sense insignificant because it is possessed by all objects, animate or inanimate. A stone may have a soul, but it also has a shape, and it is the shape that interests us, not the soul. Likewise, a micro-circuit may have a 'consciousness', a special sort of sub-molecular identity, but the vital factor is the way it shapes up to the job of retaining the memory of an event.

If this confidence is justified, there is of course the possibility of extra-physical immortality, a part 'consciousness' remaining in the computer in the guise of a recall assembly for ever, or at least as long as the computer lasts. And, as we shall see in due course, there is a chance that 'consciousness' might be conserved in this way, and may be a better prospect for keeping identity, in the sense of sustaining a sense of self, than subsequent transfer to another brain.

'Consciousness' is one thing, but identity is quite another. Identity is the continuity of consciousness within one person. As we shall see, it is one thing to transfer thought, but quite another to transfer self. In fact, if we are obsessed with the idea of keeping 'self' alive, as distinct from thought, we must cloak existence in a computer simulator, and not in any other person's brain. In a personal computer we should, in a very restricted sense, still be ourselves. In another brain we should be thoughts that someone else would be thinking. However, before we tackle this somewhat daunting objection to the whole exercise, let us clear a little more ground.

We come, in fact, to a set of somewhat speculative assumptions about the nature of the brain economics. Is it correct to assume that within the recipient's brain there will be circuits to spare for the transplant assembly, or will there be a need to blot out existing memories in the recipient in order to gain space?

It is probably not fair to assume, as some have done, that the existence of a brain outstation in the eye indicates that there is a shortage of space within. The siting of such outstations may be a deliberate attempt on the part of evolutional control to cut down the decision-time for visual judgments by arranging for much of the job to be done outside the skull. It is probably also true that the limitations of the brain are not set by the number of brain cells (this is immense) nor by the number of interconnecting fibres (this is colossal) nor even by the possible combinations which these allow (these are astronomical) but by problems of circuiting economics. A block of stone can yield a vast number of sculptured faces – but a sculptured stone cobweb, true to size, would be the work of a generation of craftsmen. In terms of artistic economics it is a non-starter. Similarly, one suspects that a very large amount of potential brain circuitry remains unused because of the restrictions of brain economics.

In any brain there is probably a near-infinite number of recall-assembly circuits which could be constructed; tenuous, bizarre entities perhaps, but still constructible. The problem is to guarantee their stability when constructed, and to make sure that the construction does not absorb too much effort at the expense of other more viable and useful assemblies.

The phenomenon of creativity is probably close to this, in that to be creative or original depends on an ability to hold unusual assemblies in resonance long enough for newer ideas to be generated. But in brain to brain transfer the assembly-input unit will not be interested in such marginal potentialities. It will be seeking the best and most economical fit for its recall assembly.

It has been suggested that much new work in the making up of micro-circuits might be saved if the input unit could find existing circuits that corresponded exactly in resonance patterns to the ones it intended to feed in. Unfortunately, except in job assembly circuits (those relating to voice fragments or smell models), identicals of this kind would be rare. Experiences differ from person to person despite the fact that such model fragments are organized on similar bases so that we can all identify a spoken word or common odour. They differ because experience must by necessity be different – we cannot all view the same thing from the same place at the same time. So, though the input unit may find some common mental nuts and bolts, the main job of transfer will probably entail a tremendous amount of frequency adjustments in circuits, and a forging of new connections.

This mapping of best paths and fresh circuitry will certainly take time, and probably necessitate the recipient remaining immobile and linked with the simulators, which may involve lengthy periods of unconsciousness or twilight experiences.

The further, really tough, technical problems will be to ensure that the input assembly will be maintained more or less intact, and not become a backwater assembly, thought about only very infrequently. Last but not least it ought not to be in sharp conflict or contrast with other assemblies of whatever kind.

To guarantee the first, of course, is probably impossible, at least as far as arranging for the thought pattern to be just as the donor experienced it. The brain is a dynamic entity, and recall assemblies that exist within it, whether they be constructed normally or implanted artificially, would be liable to change. The rate and extent of change may vary, of course, but it seems that change there must be. It is not difficult to understand why this should be so. The brain is a colossal self-regulating electro-chemical machine, with many tasks, some sequential, some simultaneous. In any such machine the possibility of flash-overs, affecting adjacent circuits, or frequency variations tripping off inappropriate responses, must be high. An added factor is brain economics, the ability of a complicated system to organize itself in ways that economize on time and energy, and eliminate duplication. Whether the transplanted assembly does, in fact, become a backwater, displaced from the main stream of conscious thought. will of course depend upon its relationship with other assemblies, To be mainstream, in fact, is a situation where the chances of drifting out of mind are small because the number of potential circuits for reactivation is high.

One can see also that such an interlocking state must presuppose a relatively small amount of conflict or contrast between the transplanter and the existing assemblies. This will all depend upon a great deal of preliminary work – tests of compatability, donor to recipient, studies of life styles, and much else besides.

How will the input assembly be experienced by the recipient? For a range of reasons we must adopt the view that it will not have the intricacy of interconnection with other assemblies in the recipient's brain, and therefore its elements will not be reality-testable at full range as other memory elements presumably are.

If, for example, a college lecturer fantasizes himself in the role of Jesus Christ or Oliver Cromwell, he has a whole range of recall assemblies against which to check the 'reality' of this fantasy. Of course, unless he is very concerned about his sanity he does not consciously perform this reality check each time he drifts into fantasy. Nevertheless, it is presumably being performed for him on an automatic basis, and it is probably a sort of statistical machine, weighing probabilities. For example, it weighs the probabilities that having a whole range of recall assemblies arranged around, say, a somewhat reclusive petit bourgeois childhood and a subsequent academic career, he should now take on the identity reality of a seventeenth-century politician-cum-soldier, and finds the chances negligible. Similarly, unless the input assembly's items are in very close conformity with existing assemblies, so as to satisfy the statistical machine, they will be judged improbable, and *thought about as fantasies*.

But they will be fantasies of an unusual kind, because true fantasy arises from memory as a kind of creative combination of experiences, a sort of very flexible recall assembly without the check of reality. And so they will be rather more than fantasy. They will be identified as alien thoughts.

The distinction between memory and fantasy is of course very fine, and yet in normal minds this distinction is maintained by the reality-testing apparatus previously described. We have little information about this apparatus. We know, for example, that it may fail. Normally, when memories are very distant and hazy – say those of childhood recalled in late adult life – confusion is likely to be between fantasy and memory of similar ages. Fresh fantasy, in other words, seldom replaces old memory, but old memory is vulnerable to old fantasy. When current fantasy replaces memory then we may have a situation of insanity, and in these cases reality is being blocked not so much by time, and the fact that time sweeps away evidence, but by a formidable assault of the fantasy systems upon the checking mechanisms.

We now have to face again the question of the extent to which identity can be conserved by these sorts of transfers. We can visualize the situation when the recipient brain has received the assembly implant which has been selected and tailored to fit an existing mental structure. Presumably within the design has been built some form of inducement which will increase the assembly's chances of being thought about. And conceivably this might put a premium on the selection of assemblies for implants having a strong pleasurable or instinctual flavour: say, an assembly of a prolonged sexual relationship.

But identity is not a tag which can be transferred. Identity is the chain of experience, occurring within one focus, or within one body. It is the continuity of that experience which provides the feel of identity; in fact it comes by practice or habit as a useful way of linking an unending set of experiences.

How does memory or the sequence of memories, natural or implanted, relate to identity? We can look at the problem in four situations. The first would be the fact that I recall some event I have observed, found significant and wished to remember. The second would be your recall of a given event, which you found significant and wished to remember. The third would be your recall of an event previously observed by me, but now implanted in you. And the fourth would be my event, recalled by you, relating and identifying itself within me.

The first two situations are of course the commonplace, and save for one question act as the foundation for the logical structure. This vital question is: does a recall assembly have any overriding sense of self? Does it, in effect, recognize itself as part of a continuity which calls itself a self? This is not the same as the recall assembly's own identity. Presumably there is a sense in which it has one of these – even though it may be not an assembly summoned very often, which lies about in a great state of dispersal. But there is no reason to suppose that a recall assembly has an overriding sense of self, and if, of course, it does not have it in the normal state it can scarcely be expected to suddenly demonstrate in the abnormal. In other words, an implant recall assembly will not conserve original (donor) identity, it will reinforce the identity of the recipient in the same way as the recipient's other pre-implant assemblies.

At this point a serious objection intrudes. If the transplanted recall assembly has no self-reference, no knowledge of itself as itself, and blends within the sequential 'consciousness' of the recipient, what kind of inducement does it offer to a would-be donor to allow himself to be tampered with in this way? What will he get out of it? Will the process offer any more concrete prospect of immortality than, say, the situation in which he might be remembered by someone else, or conceivably the faint possibility that some elements of his identity might be inherited by his children? Does it equal in inducement the promises of spiritual immortality held by some religions?

There is no doubt at all that, for those who equate immortality with a sustained opportunity to go on savouring their own identity, incorporation offers very little. And there is little doubt also that, as far as one can test opinion, immortality means just that.

But 'as far as we can test opinion' is a significant phrase. The idea of incorporation seems to involve some presupposition of conflict, and yet, as far as this study goes, this does not seem to be a likely consequence. It is possible therefore that prejudice against incorporation might be based upon a misunderstanding, a failure to realize that although the donor's identity disappears the recipient's identity is supplemented and therefore subtly changed.

This is not to be compared with the situation of being remembered by somebody else. For a start, there is no certainty of being remembered; furthermore, the memory would not be in the terms of the subject's own experience but would be through the process of the memorizer's senses. A recall assembly transplant offers the certain prospect that some element of oneself, an experience that one has made one's own, will be implanted, and will influence the behaviour of another surviving person.

The immortality offered by religions or cults is personal, of course, but unguaranteed, and spiritual or psychic, not physical. Only the inherited identity elements, in fact the actual genetic transmission of memories equals the incorporation technique in scope. Unfortunately, the evidence for this is, and may well remain, very speculative.

Looked at from the standpoint of the individual the incorporations technique with all its inadequacies may well seem the best substitute for personal immortality obtainable. But it will not, of course, satisfy the other important problem of immortality, that of bereavement grief felt by relatives. Relatives will not be able to relocate their spouses, children, parents, etc., within the incorporation, and resume death-interrupted relationships as if there had been no interruption. As far as relations or friends are concerned, almost all the satisfaction of these relationships would be experienced by the donor before death. After death and in a new identity there will be a new merged existence for the dead donor, but no sense of personal gain. For the friends or relations this will not represent an identifiable reincarnation, and consequently there will not be the social difficulties that their 'cleaving to the recipient' could create.

6

Remorseless Numbers

By seeking too much freedom, man may sink into the most abysmal forms of slavery. And yet it is freedom that the immortalist seeks. Will he be able to so arrange his world so that, having successfully conquered death, he is not overwhelmed by the consequences?

The title of this section is remorseless numbers, and certainly numbers in a immortalist world would be remorseless. This adjective may seem surprising and extravagent to those who have only had opportunities to witness gentle numerical progressions in their lives, and do not conceive of any situation more drastic. But the concept of quick and violent numerical increase, dependent on familiar mathematical bases but showing the power of geometrical increase, is a frightening novelty. Such increases will be clearly demonstrated in this section.

It has been calculated, and this gives us an idea of the extraordinary capacity of geometrical increase, that if life had been unnegated from the beginning, that is, if it had not been accompanied by death, we should by now be part of a solid ball of flesh expanding into the universe at a speed approaching that of light. This is a fantastically qualified speculation, for reasons that we need not explore, but it serves to show the magnitude of the numerical forces that lie in wait for the unwary immortalist.

But let us confine ourselves then in this discussion to the United Kingdom, admitting right from the beginning several qualifications to the arguments developed, and take these base-line facts obtained in 1970:

Total Population U.K.	*Area of U.K. per Person*	*Daily Food Ration* (Calculated on U.K. total carbohydrate output per person)
53,788,000	1·007 acres	2·5 lb

It must be admitted from the start that these figures do not look very exciting; more important they are not in themselves cause for alarm. The *per capita*, daily ration is adequate (it becomes a little more exciting if there is some exchange of carbohydrates for animal feeding stuffs) the amount of space is generous (although we make poor use of it) and we are not on the edge of either cannibalism or elbow-jostling.

Now let us do some very crude projections. Let us assume an immediate breakthrough in longevity techniques which offer a two-hundred-year life span to every living person in the United Kingdom. Let us also assume that the production of carbohydrates rises by one per cent for the next 100 years from a base date of 1970. Let us further assume that nobody dies except by accident or suicide, and that the birth rate remains the same.

The last assumption is, in fact, the most dangerous of all, because as we shall see birth rate is a very flexible entity depending upon many factors. These can be nutritional, social, medical, etc., etc., but from the standpoint of this study they principally involve the number of child-bearing women in the population, and the length of their reproductive lives.

As we can see the position changes abruptly in the hundred years that separate us from 2070.

Total Population U.K.	*Area of U.K. per Person*	*Daily Food Ration* (Calculated on U.K. total carbohydrate output, per person)
148,788,000	0·3 acre	1·3 lb

Now the figures look much more menacing. The population has increased threefold, the personal area has shrunk by an equal amount but, most imposing of all, despite a steady increase in food production the daily ration has gone below subsistence level.

Of course after 2070 the population begins to experience its first deaths when all our current centenarians start to die at the end of their extended life programme. And there is one point to remember. It is that within these figures we have assumed that the reproductive life of women has not lengthened by a day, despite the fact that all growing generations are living two-and-a-half times as long.

In fact, if we allow the slightest extension of reproductive life, all the deaths that might take place after 2070 would be a cobweb against the enormous upsurge in numbers that would almost immediately occur.

We need complex mathematics and a computer to calculate projections of this kind. The reason for this is that as soon as any increase in the reproductive life is allowed, it is immediately translated into a higher birthrate of children who will, if they are girls, also have longer reproductive lives. This again is translated into a higher birthrate, and a consequent increase in the number of women with greater opportunities of producing children, and so on, and so on. There is another point which should now be made, which probably has not come out fully in the previous statistics, although it is of particular significance to them. It is the problem of overlapping lives.

A glance at the population diagram (Fig. 8) will show the force of this argument fully. If two persons start a family with a single child, and one outlives the moment of a grandchild starting a family, then at that point the population has doubled even though the original pair of spouses did not replace itself numerically. Thus it can be seen that the problem of population is not simply a problem of replacement.

It is rather that at any given time age overlap means that a much bigger population is in existence than might be anticipated from simple addition and subtraction of people. Of course, huge increases in actual population would result if the generation overlap were to cover say twenty generations. In this case we could envisage the diagram extended in terms of generation sequence across and down the page, so that at any given moment after say, 200 years, ten times the increase would derive from a single marriage even if every child-bearing woman were to be restricted to one child.

In fact, populations that contain large numbers of people with extended lifespans will demonstrate the factors of overlapping lives and probably enlarged reproductive spans. It is obvious therefore that the projections that have been presented are the most optimistic we could conceive of. A more likely situation, given a much extended expectation of life together with a doubling or trebling of reproductive span, would be a colossal population explosion, occurring some time in the early part of the twenty-second century.

Any immortalist or semi-immortalist society would therefore have to make rapid decisions about its reproductive rate. And these rapid decisions would need to be accurate. First of all, any overall plan for authorized propagation would probably have to consider and account for many different aspects of an extended lifespan scheme. To begin with, there would possibly be a variety

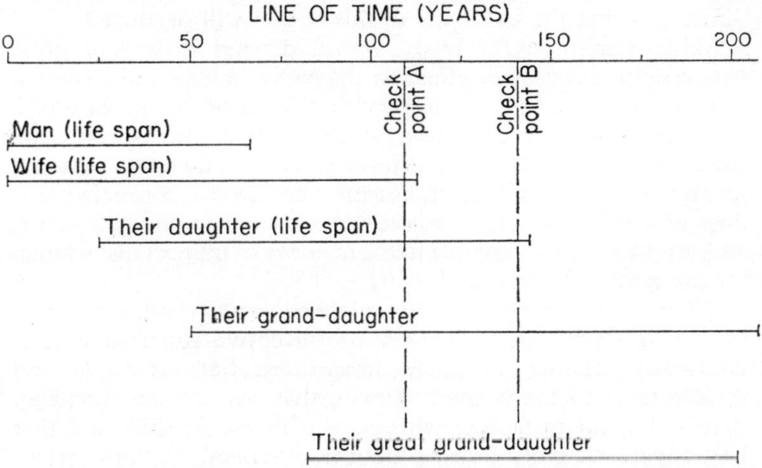

Fig. 8

of different lengths of lifespan available, ranging from the natural length (it is difficult to estimate what a 'natural' length might be) to highly unnatural spans tied to very different modes of living, involving, for instance, within one range the careful, near-immobile existence of virtual immortality, to the more carefree, less controlled existence that might end at approximately 150 years of age.

Authorized propagation might need to take account of all such different programmes of lifespan, and the ways in which they would influence the balance of life and death. Such calculations, and they would need to be very intricate, might have to predict the effect of authorizing propagation of any given applicant in any kind of lifespan.

We can, however, assume one certainty about any such schemes of authorized propagation, namely that persons with very long lifespans, or immortalists, would be banned from reproducing children. We can assume this beyond any considerations of begetting merit, i.e. any particular characteristics which might normally be held to be of value if passed on to children. We can assume this because of the overriding force of the principle of equity, the life-for-a-life principle which will undoubtedly underpin any such new society.

And thus we can deduce a strict control of immortalist men and women, in terms of a sophisticated, fool-proof, psychopath-proof system of ensuring that the option of immortality also entails sterility. What does our experience tell us about the difficulties that the enforcing of this option will produce?

Modern methods of birth control depend to a very great extent upon a conscious effort on the part of a man and a woman to wear an appliance, obtain servicing for it or, in the case of a drug, to remember to take it at the correct, birth-preventing times. Such methods as the intra-uterine spiral do not necessarily involve quite so much effort, but this very design, consisting as it does of a relatively crude barrier device, can be uncomfortable, and might not be acceptable to the majority of immortalist women for the periods we are envisaging.

What is in fact required for 'planned' or 'exchange procreation' is a device performing a contraceptive function that is constantly reliable, of micro-dimensions, both invisible and undetectable to the woman or man, that requires no servicing, that is difficult to tamper with, save with expert skill, and that lasts a woman's child-bearing lifetime, or a man's fertility period.

Only this kind of device would answer the 'planned or exchange procreation' need, because this device would make it necessary for a man or a woman to gain official consent for the removal of the device, before they conceived a child. How far are we away from such a device, which would prevent irresponsible persons taking advantage of extended lifespans, and then giving birth to unofficial progeny?

Recently in Australia a new and very ingenious implantable pump has been designed, which will deliver to the bloodstream a minute amount of any given substance provided that substance can be reduced into liquid form. In its original model it is in the shape of a capsule with three compartments. One compartment holds the liquid to be injected, and is separated by a non-permeable membrane from a second capsule containing a dye. Adjacent to this is another compartment containing water.

Gradually, water from body fluids begins to work its way through the capsule wall and to fill up the water compartment. As it does so, it forces up the pressure of the dye compartment, and makes it bulge into the next one, containing the liquid drug. Pressure thereupon rises in this compartment, which also has rigid walls, but only to a certain level, for at a prearranged point a tiny amount of the drug leaks out through a valve into the bloodstream, and the pressure then falls. The cycle is then set to start again with water gradually working through from the first compartment, raising the pressure in the second, and consequently in the third. Now of course there are all kinds of ways of controlling the rate at which the drug leaks into the bloodstream. The initial pressure is merely a sort of sweating of water through the membrane with the rate of sweat controlled by the membrane's pores. As we have seen in other chapters, a great deal of possible lifespan extension depends upon membranes such as these, and much research is currently being put into them. It may be possible to build a membrane which is electrically controlled, which has in simple terms, the dimension of its pores magnetically determined, and therefore the rate at which it will pass water. This introduces the possibility of still further refinements for the Australian device, because the effects of the drug in the bloodstream could be measured, and the results fed back to control the membrane's porosity. In this way not even the minutest amount of the drug could be over-administered, and a big saving in drug volume made.

This is one broad area of technique which might become vital for long-term birth control. There is another called the soluble capsule method which has, at this point of time, equally good potential for development. The most sophisticated variety of this technique depends on the fact that different chemicals dissolve capsules at different rates. Encapsulating such a chemical (say a specially prepared contraceptive mixture) inside a small sac, immediately starts off a reaction, which causes the formation of a solid mass of chemical material, half mixture and half sac. If this sac is placed inside the human body, then a second reaction starts when the body chemicals start to dissolve the already half-dissolved sac. The retaining wrapper's dissolution makes it possible for a readily available but low concentrate of the original chemical to be leached off gently into the blood stream.

This is the sophisticated form of the soluble capsule, but there is a simpler variety which may, however, lend itself to even greater elaborations, when some of the more intricate mechanisms of the body are understood. A capsule or sac containing chemicals which will not dissolve its case, but whose case is soluble by body chemicals, will probably split open at a predetermined time, dependent on its thickness, and release all its chemical contents into the bloodstream. There will be minimal control of release; as soon as the capsule ruptures, the contents will disperse. But of course by the placing of multi-capsules with differing times to point of rupture, a complete orchestration of release could be obtained. It may be possible to time the release to precise limits, and thereby fit the right kind of chemical to the particular need of the body at any given moment.

All these developing techniques open quite a different view on the problems of mass, and more important, involuntary birth control. With their aid society need no longer be dependent on self-administration. It may well possess a very precise instrument which can be used in conjunction with extended lifespan programmes of greater or lesser scope.

With the aid of computers a most accurate prediction and linkage of general birth rate and specific individual birth control will probably soon be developed. In individual human terms this will have certain fairly rigid consequences. We can speculate on some of these later on, but let us now deal with further methods of control.

It is likely that all would-be immortalists, or seekers after extended lifespans, would attend clinics for maintenance or servicing, and probably have to make these attendances according to a regular schedule. This would offer all the scope necessary for installing the necessary birth-control implant. The capsules or miniature pumps could be introduced into the system painlessly, by techniques that would make it very difficult for them to be tampered with by amateur surgeons. One can visualize sites being chosen behind ribs or beneath breast bones, places which should be very difficult to reach without appropriate instruments and surgical expertise.

And we can also visualize special sealing devices which would make tampering clearly detectable. For example, if a capsule had been illicitly squeezed, and thus forced to liberate its chemical in one single spurt, it might be possible to test its envelope for burstage or strong seepage and to compare it with the natural rupture caused by chemical action. Then again if the capsule or pump were to be illicitly removed, but replaced for the clinic visit, it might be possible to design a very special capsule introducer, non-possession of which would assuredly mean that, in illicit extraction or in replacement, some discernable damage would be done to the capsule.

There is of course another possible method of birth control for which some of the existing technology now exists. This is the notion of mass-medication, the control of disease by means of treating some substance in universal use like air or water with a drug that reaches all members of a given population in a standard dose. Such a method is at present in use for two sorts of disease, the special civilization-induced disease of rotting teeth for which the mass medicine is fluoride, and the group of water-borne diseases of which cholera is the most notorious, where the preventative is chlorine. There are well tried and standard procedures for introducing both these chemicals to water supplies, and since water is the only controllable substance that everybody has to ingest a certain quantity of, every day, it provides a standard dose, tailored to a general need.

It might well be possible to introduce birth-control chemicals to public water supplies. One specific problem, however, might be the physiological reaction of the male portion of the population to what would be for them an unnecessary, but compulsory, daily dose of birth-control hormone, but if this difficulty were to be overcome then a very flexible and easily workable system for mass birth control would result. The way in which mass birth control might be organized on this basis would certainly give an opportunity for irresponsible persons to avoid their daily or twice daily quota of prophylactic chemical by arranging their own private water supplies. It might therefore be necessary to plan for the prophylactic to carry with it some extra chemical essential to the life-extension process. In this combination system one could envisage all those who were anxious to have an extended lifespan attending servicing or maintenance clinics at specified intervals. But the treatment they would receive at such clinics would not of itself be sufficient to guarantee extended life. For an absolute guarantee they would have to absorb a regular supply of what we could call a catalysing chemical, which would be obtainable only from the same source as the prophylactic additive, namely the water supply. It would, needless to say, be technically impossible, without very expensive and sophisticated equipment to separate the two chemicals within one supply, and thus all who wanted to take full advantage of the life-extension service would be obliged to absorb the prophylactic as well. There would be two categories of people in the immortalists society, then – those who had opted out of extended life, and who would presumably in recognition of this be allowed an antidote to the prophylactic and thus permitted to propagate, and those on various life-span extensions who would be permanently sterile, or permitted, at best, some carefully calculated period of fertility in which they might conceive.

All this speculation about immortalists having to bow to a kind of regime of biological control does give a picture of a society under some degree of coercion. To what extent this would diminish enthusiasm for immortality it is difficult to say without knowing the future importance of a future parental role. But it is clear that even currently man plays many different roles with varying amounts of significance, never being completely restricted, whatever place in the pecking order he may occupy.

We have not, for example, touched on the economic role, with the immortalist as mercantilist. It is interesting that when we do, in fact, move into this field, we see the spectre of geometric increase immediately in front of us, as if it were waiting for the approach of immortality to rouse it. Nowhere is this spectre more distinct than when the immortalist is seen as investor.

The kind of investment power that an immortalist might wield can be astonishing when represented in quite simple terms. Let us assume that an immortalist with a 700-year lifespan has invested £100 at 6 per cent per annum, compound interest, and leaves the sum to accumulate for his entire life span. The table of accumulation is as follows:

Time Elapsed in Years	*Sum Accumulated*
50	£1,842
100	£33,930
200	£11,510,000
500	£450,000,000,000,000
700	£52,000,000,000,000,000,000

The figure at 500 years is, in literal terms, 450 million million pounds – half a billion pounds, in other words. The accumulation at 700 years is even more astounding. There are, in fact, 18 zeros behind the initial 52 in the table. In literal terms this sum is 52 million million million pounds, which is not contractible in any meaningful way, and is in excess, in sterling terms, of the total annual world gross product since computation began. We can, in fact, make some predictions about the economic life of a semi-immortalist society. The first of these is that if the present structure of capitalism survives the stresses of the transitional phase from a mortal to partially immortal society, we can expect a very sharp division in economic power between those living a normal and those living an abnormal lifespan. The table shows the accumulation of capital on an initial sum of £100 invested at 6 per cent interest over selected periods of time, As we can see, the capital appreciation is enormous, and would put the investing immortalist in an unassailable position vis-à-vis his mortal neighbour.

It would be unwise to assume, however, that the traditional financial structure would serve the transitional phase. If we want another example of how sharp the financial stresses during this period might be, we need only begin to speculate on another aspect of contemporary capitalism, the life and annuity policy. The mind boggles at the strain which would be placed upon the financial balance of life and annuity policy funds, by sudden and unanticipated increases in lifespan among policy holders. Obviously this method of investment (since this is all life and annuity policies really are) could not continue as we at present have it.

We can almost certainly assume a rigid legal framework designed to limit the scope of the immortalist in gaining political and financial advantages over his normal lifespan contemporary. It is possible to envisage several sorts of controls on immortalists which would act in this way. A very rigorous reversion code might be followed with particular reference to property and wealth. An immortalist might not be allowed to amass wealth beyond a set figure, or after a certain time. He might be required to hand back to a central property pool, or make over to a common fund, wealth that he had accumulated beyond a given limit.

At the same time one can predict a certain traditionalist strengthening of generational ties on the part of the non-immortalist section of the population. Being in the position of having to co-exist with a group that has unlimited time at its disposal would be bound to make the non-immortalist cling more tightly to his own accumulated wealth, and ponder most deeply upon the way in which he might ensure that when he passed it on it was not added to the wealth of those to whom the making of legacies and bequests was meaningless.

Economically speaking, we would expect the immortalist to be considerably constrained in certain fields. If a modified capitalism with its political structure continued, it would be altogether impossible for immortalists as a group to be involved in lending money for long periods. This would obviously exclude them from much investing activity, but it would not necessarily keep them from becoming entrepreneurs with much borrowing capacity. In this field unlimited time, though conferring some advantage, would not, little by little, make this advantage overwhelming. In any case it is likely that, however employed, an immortalist would need to be a person who made job changes – and not necessarily because of boredom. (The boredom of an immortalist is an old canard, presupposed on the boring existences of many naturals. The immortalist with a normal memory span might well be bored, like naturals, but in respect of his longer life this would not make for more boredom, because he would not remember it, and would not obviously ask his memory machine to recall it.)

Much of the job-changing of the immortalist would be in the nature of necessity. He would be around just too long for the tastes of many naturals, who would see him unchanged throughout their youth, maturity and old age. And although his continuity might be valued in some contexts, in others familiarity would eventually breed contempt.

It is not easy to gauge the mutual attitudes of immortalist and natural man. Both would be likely to have a considerable amount of ambivalence towards each other, since there would be, if not actual ambivalence, considerable paradox involved in both life styles. In addition much would depend upon the numerical strengths of the two groups. But the natural man might regard the other as self-indulgent, seeing the immortalist as having chosen to deny potential progeny the right to life, and mortal man the right to extend his family as he might wish. He might at the same time envy the immortalist's boldness in challenging fate in quite so conclusive a manner, his independence of mind, and his self-sufficiency. He might see him as a threat, the tremendous continuity of the immortalist's existence, even when hedged about with various restrictions both legal and physical, making the permanence of his own institutions seem fragile. He would certainly envy the immortalist his avoidance of a personal decision about death, particularly as the end of a natural lifespan would probably, owing to the progress of medical technology, have some of the elements of a suicidal act about it. In turn the immortalist might despise the natural man for his timidity. He might detect, or imagine, a 'life martyrdom' quality about the natural man's approach to the mysteries of existence, as though the natural man were desiring a certain sacrificial satisfaction from not having chosen immortality, a quality he might find particularly objectionable. He might envy the natural man his relative freedom from continuous clinical supervision, the conclusive nature of his relationship with both conditions of mankind, and his independence of memory machines. He might at one and the same time disdain the instinctual thrills of the natural man's life and hanker after them. There might be an element of anxiety in his attitude. He might regard himself as a rationalist, opposed by the emotional mind in respect of the very *raison d'être* of his existence, and vulnerable to a movement to regularize the life/death pattern of the world to fit the emotional needs of natural man. Indeed, he might see his existence being one of restricted horizons, opposed constantly by an unrestricted yearning for fecundity on the part of natural man.

It is not easy to predict the extent to which the immortalist would be regarded as a mysterious being. There is often a parallel drawn between the awe of the mediaeval peasant for the priestly arts, and the bewilderment of the electronically ignorant faced with the intricacies of television. It may well be that the emotion involved in both cases is similar.

Of course, there are circumstantial differences. Both priest and peasant were, in purely spiritual terms, on a similar level of ignorance; the power of the priest's office created the necessary amount of 'distance' to sustain the mystery. The immortalist would be of a different order of priesthood, a priesthood which would probably clearly understand its own strengths and limitations, even though much of what sustained it would be completely incomprehensible to the majority of persons who had everyday contact with it.

The immortalist might therefore be placed in the position of a half man, half god, at least as far as some of the population were concerned. It is important to see that the engineering, even in this non-deliberate way of man's semi-divinity, might have significant consequences for the concepts of good and evil, as these might be then defined.

Immortalists might have to take upon themselves some aspects of collective resentment, or guilt, as well as the role of being the personification of goodness and truth. Of course, there might be many of them, a factor which might lessen their importance as semi-deities to some degree. But it would not eliminate it.

The one major difference would be in the ascription of guilt. As the immortalist does not die, the notion of the death of a deity which functions as a kind of expiation or ransom for the collective wickedness of mankind would not apply. But there is a possible outcome to this that might not be quite so happy for immortalists. If a god did not die, and rid believers of their guilt, believers might take the expiatory law into their own hands, and kill him. They might do this even though they had accepted much of the immortalist's super-rational morality as their own. For the immortalists would undoubtedly break up any lingering belief in an absolute, cosmological standard for good and bad. From their vantage point they would be capable of a long view of the consequences of actions. They would be able to assess with much subjective experience whether the outcome of a given action might be to the general betterment of the greatest number or not. This would give them a certain cachet, overriding the limited experience of the natural man.

And, of course, in terms of the consequences of actions, the immortalist would be far from academically concerned. For he or she would live to see the working out of good and evil. And this also would add its own particular weight to the immortalist's moral influence – indeed, in matters which concern the distant future, their judgment would be irresistible.

This aside, the immortalist might still be precariously placed. To have a demi-god so near to hand might be too convenient a situation for the vengeful natural man to resist.

There would, of course, be many similarities between the minds of immortalists and those of natural men. They would have been designed on the same jig, so to speak, with similar cognitive, and to a large extent emotional processes, so that communication between them in many respects would be easy. But the immortalist and the natural might not entirely share each other's thinking. There might be gaps and blockings which would force them apart.

Specifically they would not share the same neuroses, and the feelings which may underpin those neuroses might not be easily conveyed. It might for example, be impossible for an immortalist to convey to a natural the impact of extra-dimensional anxiety, that sudden loosening of the boundaries of the self, which would afflict some of those who knew they would not die. The immortalist would undoubtedly have a different concept of time so that much of the neurotic doings of normal man would seem ludicrous. Anxieties which related to machines natural man would know something of, but they would be of trifling size by comparison with the fears of a man whose past was organized for him within a massive memory store, and whose future depended upon the intricate workings of mechanisms that surveyed and controlled every system in his body.

That there might well be relationships need not be doubted. But these relationships would exist in two forms of reference, unlimited and limited time, and this duality would cause its own specific stress. From the standpoint of natural man or woman, there would be the ever-present contrast of life style; in their cases the contrast between relationships of the transient sort which they might have with other normal people, and the potentially everlasting relationships that immortalists might have with other fellow immortalists. They would never be able to blot out the feeling that the immortalist they loved or admired might be possessed of the memories (admittedly electronic) of people who might have been their great grandparents, and that they might have current friendships (recall of which also partly electronic) with fellow immortalists which could conceivably extend for centuries. This would serve, at one and the same time, to make their status in the natural/immortalist relationship somewhat subordinate, and sharpen up both parties' sense of its temporary nature.

It might, however, be this sharpening up and definition that time would give to the normal person's friendships that the immortalist would come to envy. Unless he picked all his acquaintances from amongst natural people he would never be able to share the totality of the temporary friendships that the natural man or woman would experience. And he might come to feel that within this unqualified totality there lay a range of emotions that he could never hope to feel.

Interesting paradoxes are continually encountered in any study of extended lifespans. In classical terms the core of these paradoxes is contained in the assertion that 'by seeking too much freedom, man falls into the basest form of slavery'. For the immortalist the desire for freedom from death and its consummation would involve not slavery, but a willingness to subordinate oneself to a life which was computer-directed, at least to some extent, and in which some natural desires would have to be restrained.

And of course this restraint would involve not only the immortalist. It would be in a sense multi-lateral, for the man or woman living a normal lifespan would be also tied in various ways. The immortalist would probably never be able to conceive or beget children. And because of this choice of the immortalist, the man or woman who did not desire immortality would also probably be restricted in begetting or procreating. But there would be a moral problem as well, and this would involve both natural man and natural woman, and their immortalist counterparts. The easiest way for an immortalist man to beget a child would not be for him to impregnate an immortalist woman. For this would mean a double deceit; he would have to choose a natural woman, since only one deceit would then be necessary.

One can envisage certain tensions within the immortalist group. Some of these people might well feel the lack of a formal hierarchy, in the sense that no immortalist would appear significantly older than any other, which in itself might intensify the kind of rivalries that a group ordered by age could avoid. Then, of course, the physical fact of their being in so narrow an age range, and therefore likely to have ambitions in common, might mean more jostling, a sharper struggle to share the spoils.

Of course, too much must not be made of these particular idiosyncrasies. There is no doubt that rivalry is sharpened in normal groupings by time, and the fear that leaving the initiative to someone else temporarily may be to abdicate from events for good. Time as a spur would not be a meaningful concept to the immortalist. There would always be enough and to spare, and in substitution for all those warnings about the domination of time, the immortalist might comfort himself with the wry assurance that 'everything comes to him who waits'. Waiting would, of course, be the only problem for him.

The other point is that we ought not necessarily to assume that the most important social groupings would be composed entirely of members of one type. Mixed groupings would be likely also, and within mixed groupings there might be opportunities for immortalists to encounter the kinds of hierarchies and multiple roles that might be absent from their own groups. We can also predict that immortalists would experience with other immortalists a relationship that would be exclusively theirs, in the sense that it did not have a parallel, could not have a parallel, anywhere outside their own time scale. This would be the phenomenon of the deferred relationship, the deliberate decision, mutual or non-mutual, to put off the beginning of relationships for a specified or non-specified time.

We can think of all sorts of reasons for such deferments. A blocking circumstance is the most obvious – with immortalists as with natural men 'it will be as well to be off with the old love before one is on with the new', but this, of course, is in the range of the commonplace. Much more interesting might be the prospect of a deliberate tailoring of observed needs to organizable or developable skills – such as when an immortalist man saw that his potential immortalist beloved admired such and such a skill or felt comfortable in such and such a circumstance – and deliberately set out to provide the conditions under which their relationship might develop most fruitfully. Immortalists might also be able to arrange sequential relationships, developing in special ways with suitable partners, the better to satisfy other persons in a future sequence.

It is possible therefore that because of the special nature of some of the feelings that immortalists would have, and the seeming impossibility of conveying the meaning of those feelings to naturals, a kind of special jargon would develop between immortalists to enable them to intercommunicate. And this would have to be a very special jargon indeed, since in the normal order of things jargon, though a convenience for some, is explicable to many, given time. But the meaning of immortalist jargon would be quite inexplicable to the natural man, because the natural would not share parts of immortalist's feelings which underpinned it.

And by the same token, this incapability of the natural man to understand the immortalist might mean that when the immortalist became disturbed, and needed a counsellor or even (if such methods were still in vogue) a psychotherapist, he or she would have to depend upon fellow immortalists, appropriately qualified, not only in terms of psychological expertise, but also in capacity to feel similarly.

Such sympathy might mean that at significant, though not necessarily frequent (since immortalists will clearly know the consequences of their immortalist choice) stressful times in their lives, there would be a heightening of mutual relationships between immortalists to the exclusion of natural society.

We might imagine that immortalists, being the beneficiaries of a most sophisticated medical technology, would themselves be in the forefront of development and innovation in the technical field. But on the contrary they might turn out to be conservative. To begin with, theirs would be a delicately balanced state of being, liable to be pushed out of its precise tuning by environmental changes which would have little significant effect on natural man. This would make them very resistant to untried mechanical innovation with unpredictable effects. But then, of course, they would have less of the pressures of time to push them towards innovation; nor would they, if they became ingrouped, be capable of much originality, there being an absence of the catalysing force of fresh minds breaking into old groupings.

And we can anticipate that in respect of the technology that kept them what they were, they would be immensely cautious, pressing constantly for the control and maintenance of the immortalizing machines to be in the hands of immortalists like themselves, so that their futures might not be jeopardized by the whims of other beings.

What must be the final verdict on the immortalists and the society in which they would live? It would certainly not be the Armaggedon that many fear. Instead we can foresee a world of fascinating and intricate differences between men, with all the intellectual and moral activity that an ultimate choice between life and death creates. We can see man forced for the first time to take full responsibility for himself, to have and, if he is rational to hold, levering himself up out of slime, remodelling himself anew from mud and flame and finally, in a high sanctuary, becoming a god.

7

Gods Themselves

Why should man desire immortality? When we ask this question of ourselves it seems at first to carry more than a normal load of man's wilfulness and arrogance, indeed it seems to imply a kind of insolence, even in the asking.

And yet when we examine the nature of life, the question loses this initial, man-slanted, man-motivated quality. Life itself is, on the best evidence, not immortal. It is also very clearly not the same thing at all as inanimate matter, which is slowly simplifying. Life is constantly renewing itself, striving to keep itself going in a world of steady simplification by taking inanimate matter and using it to maintain itself, in a kind of fluctuating battle, the skirmishes of which are births and deaths.

And it is surely not too fanciful to suggest that if there is a battle, life may eventually triumph, not in the precarious sense in which we see it at present, but in a total, unconditional victory. In this war man may be life's ultimate weapon. He may be designed to make himself and life immortal, the necessary skills and motivations having been built into him. If this is the case then all his myths and fantasies of immortality may be in the nature of necessary rehearsals for an as yet unrealistic, but eventually to be realized, ultimate transformation.

The trouble with an argument of this kind is that it is as devastating as it is speculative, devastating to the notion of man as a free agent. It keeps its grip even if we try to discover the main motives for immortality-seeking. Our life is an uncertain existence, for reasons which may appear to lie within our own control. We can specify the risk to our species (and indeed to all other species) of death or sterilization from nuclear warfare, but at the very moment when we are questioning the morality of doing something as drastic as making ourselves immortal, because we fear the consequences of our own actions, we begin to doubt whether we really are responsible for our own actions, and whether our desire to deal out utter death is not as preordained as our desire to perfect an utter life.

If, however, seeking to justify immortality bids we search for clear non-man motivated reasons for immortality striving, we do not necessarily have to look within ourselves. At any time, the astrophysicists tell us, the earth could be struck by a colossal blast of radiation from the sun, which would kill or sterilize all life. At any time, according to the epidemiologists, a mutant virus could sweep through the world's population, slaughtering such an enormous proportion of the breeding or breedable generations that the human race would become extinct.

But quite apart from these speculative nightmares, there is one other excellent justifiable reason why man might be expected to seek immortality. It is because he cannot remain as he is. He cannot remain for much longer in a state of indecisive limbo, because he has now reached the stage when he has become too cynical and too sophisticated for his own peace of mind. He no longer believes that he in some way deserves death as a kind of punishment for his ancestral crimes, and he has got rid of the satisfying, original sin and redemption myths which at one and the same time explained the necessity for death and offered a heavenly reward for a life of instinctual restriction. As far as he is concerned, that computer of excellence in the sky against which his life was formerly to be judged has broken down.

There was a sense in which all the sin, redemption, God and computer-in-the-sky mythology was a kind of statement of docility, a charter of acceptance. But man was never very good at docility, even as it related to the way he adapted to the physical world in which he found himself – he rapidly set about changing it. Now matters have developed so that not only does he not accept the world in which he lives, he no longer accepts himself as he is. He has grown too big for his spiritual boots.

It is useless deploring the situation, for things are not likely to change. Man is extremely restless, dissatisfied and not at all to be soothed. No soother is in fact in sight. He is almost unsoothable by definition. And his very restlessness is dangerous, dangerous to his survival.

But if he has failed to come to terms with his inadequacy, will he be able to come to terms with adequacy? If he becomes immortal because he cannot stand the impotence and uncertainty of mortality, will he be more content with his lot when he is potent and certain? Will the miseries of potency and certainty be of the same quality as those he experiences in his present form? Although we can say little about them, one thing is clear. It is better to be miserable in potence and certainty, for at least man's new powers may give him another option, the opportunity to tackle constructively the fresh things he may become miserable about. If on the other hand he finds he cannot cope with the miseries of immortality, he can always destroy himself.

Throughout the previous discussions we have been speculating on man in various states of physical change, without specifying the extent to which these may make him a different sort of psychological being. There is, of course, a good reason for this tactic. It is that though we can talk about physical changes in extended lifespans in relatively clear terms, we cannot do the same for psychological consequences. Such consequences follow as supplementary speculations.

Nevertheless, although we are forced to speculate in this sense, a system can still be followed. We can take four varieties of mental functioning – Memory, Perceptions, Affects and Compulsions – and test each within the fresh context of physical immortality to see how each performs. Before the sequence starts it ought to be pointed out that the functions chosen are somewhat arbitrary, but that the order of the sequence is deliberate, in that Memory is the lynch-pin function around which the remainder revolve. This technique makes the discussion much more variable than it might be with another sequence, but since reordering is one method of discovery, it may be viewed as a benefit rather than a liability.

There are at present several theories of memory, or rather recall, which are not mutually exclusive, and which may at some point in the future be combined as stages in a larger theoretical process. Whether they concentrate on the problems of storage (memories dispersed in molecular-size codes throughout the brain) or of retrieval (lifting out an appropriate memory at the right time) they do not offer any solutions to the problem of storage during a very long lifespan. Commonsense would suggest that there is a limit to the amount of material that can be retained in the memory and, even if there were to be an attempt to pack more in by infinitesimal fragmentation, this would eventually lead to a breakdown of recall because the process of retrieval would become too complex.

With this in mind we must take a close look at the halt situation, and speculate on how far this stabilizing of all the electrical and chemical processes of the body might affect the memory function.

It is just possible that in a situation where ageing is stopped the stability would be so precarious that any non-cyclical change of a chemico-molecular kind might cause the organism to become unstable, and consequently to begin to deteriorate. Such a halt would require an absolute regularity and predictability on the part of all body systems. Its effect in terms of memory might be very significant indeed.

To begin with, it is supposed that long-term memory is an electro-chemical process involving changes in the molecular structure of the brain. An ultra-stable state would freeze those systems into permanent rigidity, and they would therefore be unable to take in and incorporate new experiences. Short-term memory is believed to be dominantly electrical, however, with little chemical dependence, and therefore an immortalist might keep his short-term memory. This, however, has only a limited duration – in some people a matter of seconds.

This would mean that the immortalist was mnemonically linked to a past which could not be either forgotten or added to, which was in constant relation to a changing world, but was not changed by it. The immortalist would be able to retain new experiences mnemonically for a matter of seconds (and of course indefinitely if they were recorded) but they would not be able to interact with the corpus of his past experiences.

We can however envisage a much more convenient form of halt, which might leave the normal mnemonic systems intact, and working in their usual ways. In other words, the immortalist would possess normal long- and short-term memory. When we consider the adjective 'normal' in relation to memory we do, in fact, somewhat outstrip our knowledge, in that we know a good deal about the length of short-term memory but very little of the mechanism of either. One thing is fairly certain, though. Normal memory span would not be long enough for the immortalist.

Let us assume that the normal long-term memory span lasts about a century from birth, after which time memories, acquired in the early stages of life, become hazy and more difficult to retrieve. There are, of course, no grounds for assuming that for the immortalist memory would be cut off in a neat, regular fashion – indeed the opposite would be the case. If we think of memory in its widest sense, and include skills, then there need be no reason why patterns in constant use should not be retained indefinitely. But, of course, there would be a limit to the amount of material that could be kept 'polished up' in this way, and thus gradually as time progressed longer and longer gaps would open up in the mnemonic span, and more and more would be felt to have fallen out.

Unfortunately, the social and biological conventions that protect our failing memories in mortal life (the fallibility of other people's memories; the lack of interest in other people's past, which seems irrelevant to the young; the progress of innovation, which makes large areas of memories redundant) may not operate for the immortalist.

To begin with, that aspect of the past which includes personal relationships will probably not, as at present, be comfortably consignable to limbo, because of the small chance in natural life of ever establishing old relationships – death and chance intervening. In the immortalist's world, there will always be the chance of bumping into persons 'known' more than a hundred years ago, and having to re-establish some contact with them.

It is easy enough to let laziness get in the way of speculations at this point, and to say that in such a situation some kind of balance would have to be struck between the capacity of human memory, and the trend to immediacy.

Unfortunately despite this evasion it is only too clear what man's attitude would be, when confronted with the necessity to obtain the advantages of an unlimited memory span. He would immediately seek a memory substitute in the shape of a memory machine.

At this point an exquisite dilemma inserts itself. It is not so much the fact that immortal man will be forced to objectify his past, in other words to see it in display form presented to him by some machine. It is rather that the very necessities of the system, the bulk of the data to be stored, and the speed with which large quantities of it may need to be scanned (some decisions may still need to be made with speed) will necessitate some degree of autonomy, or decision-making responsibility being given to the machine.

Of course, if we revert for a moment to the predicament of the *immediate memory* man in this situation, here we have an even more exquisite problem, because the 'immediate memory' man would have no more than his immediate memory span to scan machine displays, and would therefore be assigning even more decision-making responsibility to his machine.

Whichever model we take, then, whether it be normal or frozen, we can see significant changes for the immortalist. These must of necessity require a much greater dependence on machinery, so that the important decision for the immortalist will be to balance the advantage of a comprehensive mechanical memory with the disadvantages of assigning some personal decision-making responsibility to a machine.

Of course it is not all debt and difficulty. Apart from suicide, which like the choice of natural death would still be a leap into the void, we can also visualize a most fascinating notion of death, but in a form which would permit man all the satisfaction, but none of the woes. The immortalist would be able to command forgetfulness, for himself, by manipulating his machine. In respect of individuals and events best forgotten, he would be able to erase them at will. And if he could persuade other people who might also have been involved to do the same, he would do death's work more effectively than death. He who controls the present controls the past in respect of events entirely, but in respect of persons probably alive, only partially. And yet to have an entirely fresh encounter with a hated person 'killed' mnemonically is easier than remembering him, and easier than meeting him as remembered. It is only in a very limited sense that the living, who have been forgotten, still go marching around.

A frozen memory would of course have drastic implications for perception. An immortalist with such a memory would be incapable of retaining the small changes in the environment which normally are unconsciously remembered. This would cause a continuous series of fresh perceptual encounters, rather similar in sensation to the normal lifetime experience of returning to a well-remembered place after a lapse of time and finding it changed, except that for the frozen immortalist this sensation would be much more common. Thus the frozen immortalist would have a very strong incentive to keep the environment just as it was, unless, of course, he found the sensation pleasurable.

Strange though this situation might be, however, the effect of physiological halting would probably have even greater consequences for man's perception of time.

The sensation or perception of time is probably the result of a synthesis. We observe and note all the available scales for judging time's passing; the movement of clocks, the progress through the calendar, plus the cyclical variations of sun and season. We then combine this data with the facts of entropy, the processes of decay, both in ourselves and in others, and the apparently timeless experiences outside (for the rotation of a clock or the sun does not of itself imply any time lapse) and from this combination we come to a concept of time.

It is important to see therefore that the immortalist would experience no sensations of internal change as they affected him. The most that he would experience would be a gradual feeling of mnemonic distance as memories began to fade, and this would be his only subjective entropic sensation. Immortalist man would therefore be stripped of nearly all synthetic sensations of time. It is true that he would see external change. Trees would grow, and eventually fall, but these happenings would not involve him in their chronological process. They would have the same relation to him as clocks and from his vantage point, being able to see an infinite number of trees rise and fall, the same artificial significance as clocks.

But the aspect of motive must not be neglected. One very significant impulse to technological creativity is the desire to telescope time. In this cause, man destroys distance and time by speed. By the application of power he enables himself to cram a number of notional lifetimes (judged in pre-technological, historical terms) into one.

Obviously the impulse to seek even faster methods of time telescoping would weaken for the immortalist. But if time were inconsequential, in the sense of there no longer being a shortage of it, the very fact of its sudden change to surplus would create a new kind of motivation, a desire for continuous occupational/recreational variety.

Now this could be a very strong motivation indeed, and realizing its objectives not so difficult as might immediately be assumed. One great advantage, as has been pointed out, of having a machine memory covering the distant past is that one may command it to forget inconvenient facts, possibly the recollections of recreations or occupations which if allowed to come up for review might cause a sensation of boredom. It would thus be possible to uncouple a strongly permutational future (composed of combining creatively hobbies, jobs and amusements) from a permutated past, and thus to destroy the feeling of boredom.

Mortal man is time-bound, and the boundaries of time give their own special meaning as a backcloth against which the drama of life is played, establishing their own forms of dramatic convention. If the backcloth were removed man would gaze out into eternity, and the conventions would lapse. They would lapse, but soon they would be retrieved, not in the form of a new backcloth, since that would be gone for good, but in a greater strengthening of the internal rules of the drama. In fact, the drama would cease to be externally contrasted; it would become a series of games with intricate rules, each rule system acting as a kind of little universe, and attracting to itself a strong emotional commitment. Life would no longer consist of work and play, each compartmentalized. Play and the rules of play, extraordinarily strengthened, would invade all existence.

What might be the emotional effects of such experiences of timelessness? It is, of course, very difficult to be precise about these – we have no good analogies to the state within our experience. But weightlessness is probably as close as we can come to a condition in which the body's normal state of gravity relation is completely eliminated, and left to find its own equilibrium.

Weightlessness does not seem to be an alarming condition in itself. That is to say the mind does not react immediately to the weightless situation with panic, although, of course, we do not have any valid long-term experiences to judge by, and we do not know, for example, if the physiological consequences of weightlessness may not in the end generate their own special brand of anxiety as a kind of biological survival device. On the analogy then of weightlessness, and unless there are some special unknown mental consequences in being suspended in time, we may therefore anticipate no adverse emotional effects, from the personal suspension of time.

There may well be items in the credit account. One of the most important restraints on the activities of man is the limitation of time. When we say that we have not time for such and such an activity, or have gone about as far with a given scheme as time allows, we in fact have made a cost-benefit estimate, and from that estimate a decision. We have rationed activity within time, because time has definite limits for us.

The immortalist, of course, would face no such definite limits. Time would radiate out from his position in an infinite stream, and we might therefore naively suppose that his activities would not be circumscribed in any way.

Although much of the anxiety that is generated by ambition pressing against the restraints of time would, of course, disappear, it would be a mistake to think that such restraints are entirely negative in their operation, in other words, that they operate against man's interest in all respects. There may well be a sense in which just having time to do a thing provides an incentive for doing it. We shall reconsider this point in relation to innovations later.

Another perceptual feature, or at least a feature which can be identified in the perceptual/cognitive field is identity convergence. In our mortal life this term means the gradual growing together in patterns of behaviour of people whose lives are lived in very close proximity, like spouses. Of course, it is very difficult to disentangle the factors involved in this process. We must certainly bear in mind that the act of becoming spouses presupposes a good deal of previous personal similarity on the part of the people involved, and it would also be unwise to discount the influence of an environment which both by definition must share.

But when these factors have been allowed for, we are still faced with the existence of a balance of convergence, that seems to be inexplicable except by a kind of mutual shaping and conditioning process which eventually brings both personalities to a much deeper basis of common understanding. Nor does it stop at psychological convergence. Some observers have noticed that spouses or persons in spouse-like situations seem to become more alike in facial expressions. Here again we must attribute some of the observed effect to the influence of original mutual choosing – like choosing like, not only on the basis of some kind of physical similarity but perhaps also in a more complicated relationship through the picking of partners resembling mothers or fathers.

If we accept the influence of proximity as being an important factor in these convergences, there are important consequences implicit for extended lifespans. Of course, we do not know whether the states we see in normal lifetimes are capable of further convergence, or whether they are terminal. If, however, they are continually in process, so to speak, and are brought to an end only by the death of one of the partners, then the extended lifespan opens up a prospect of gradually increasing identity convergence since both partners will live much longer, or possibly be immortal.

We may speculate also on the psychological meanings of such convergences. Do they represent a benign transition from a state of self-separatism to one of self-merging, and as such are they an early manifestation of a kind of developing interpersonal paradise? Or might they be very dependent upon life stages, not developing at all if the personalities involved did not pass together through the phases of courtship, child rearing, consolidation, deterioration and death?

If they were not phase-dependent, and even if in the immortalist world there were no such role as a spouse, might we expect convergence to progress to a point when two identities would become one? Further psychological research may be able to tell us the answer to this question. It may be able to show that there are limits to the extent to which one person can become like another, that there exist built-in checks to the process going on to a final state of total identification, and that when such a checkpoint is reached, there can be no more movement.

We also, of course, do not know what effect immortality may have upon the sense of self. It is possible that there is some connection between the boundaries of the self and the knowledge that the self has mortal limits, some sort of buffer apparatus that, through the mechanisms of deterioration, preserves the uniqueness of an individual's identity. It is impossible to speculate in this area, because we have no current experiences to work with. But it is also not necessary to regard uniqueness as having an absolute value. To lose it might be an emancipation.

The immortalist might of course be emancipated in other obvious ways. First and foremost, he could be rid of his fear of death. Fearing death, and lacking the power to do anything about it, man has had to take refuge in many different sorts of evasions. He formerly gave up great quantities of his reason and emotions to self-identified prophets proclaiming various sorts of immortality, who had an unfortunate habit of publicly panicking when faced with imminent death. Such prophets talked about immortality in vague and ambiguous terms, passing themselves off, often successfully, as the special representatives of God, and therefore as possessors of occult and highly significant knowledge. Sometimes finding such prophets puzzling, and their followers dubious (they always seem to leave behind them rather less convincing models of themselves, who swiftly compensate for what they lack in charisma by a swift grasp of secular sources of power and influence) man turned to spiritualistic cults, specializing in the 'demonstration' of spiritual immortality. But all these strategies seem to have done nothing to ease his fear of death; he constantly strives for new faiths, new interpretations, falls into various sorts of apathies, or attempts to obliterate anxiety by frantic distractions, sexual or occupational.

Personal immortality will rid man of certain features of this chronic impotence. It will help him ignore the mystery-mongers with their special relationship with the Almighty, and their references to some universal moralizing machine that makes up a balance sheet of good or bad on earth. And it will strip away the cosmological and metaphysical guilts attaching to those sort of beliefs, which are so eagerly reinforced by those who profit from the reality of mortal man in mortal chains.

But as mortal man becomes emancipated so he will develop new commitments. Mortal man has a bond with the earth from which he was organized. Earth as far as we know abides, but man does not, and therefore man must feel, though he may not readily admit it, some sense of inferiority in relation to all the mighty, enduring things around and underneath him. It would be fair to postulate as the consequence of this sense of inferiority that mortal man, deeply aware of the essentially contingent and temporary nature of his life, may often either overvalue or undervalue it.

In overvaluation there may be great obsessional clinging to life, a kind of irrational indignation at the steady process of change and decay. At the other extreme we can clearly see a most depressive devaluation, very common amongst those who believe in various forms of afterlife in the non-physical sense.

One effect of immortality may be to modify man's attitude to life on earth by trimming off these extremes. For the first time man will have the power to be himself, to make his own valuation of life, and the effect may be to create between him and earth a new non-clinging, non-changing bond. This will be a relationship of equals, and the result may be that man may develop an entirely new sense of personal commitment to earth – a brother-earth philosophy of deep and abiding dimension.

Man may also come to a greater degree of self-knowledge. In a normal lifetime, unless we are especially gifted analytically, we seldom if ever come to a full understanding of the emotional mechanisms or our motivations. In the main this is due to the fact that we just do not have enough time or experience in which to explain ourselves to ourselves. Psychoanalysis may be viewed as a method of economic search, a picking out of the most significant of a lifetime's experiences for study, a telescoping of time. But formal psychoanalysis, as for that matter any systematized exposure to analysis, does not reach more than a small fraction of the population. But when experiences are unlimited even the most untutored of immortalists will need no psychoanalysis to know themselves.

These are in a sense emotional gains. By contrast to them we can identify two possible sources of anxiety. The first and most vague of these is Extra-dimensional Anxiety, which is very difficult to conceptualize, and yet might trouble immortal man. It is almost an axiom (almost, because there are certain limitations to the seeming law) that nothing is truly conceivable without the simultaneous knowledge of its negation. All the things we see in the concrete sense, all the objects of our existence, are securely fixed in the context of their non-being. That is to say if we glimpse a tree, we simultaneously have the concept, implied, though not necessarily pondered upon, of the tree being cut down, blown down, burnt or transformed into useable secondary objects, all of which would have a being, and a non-being too.

Concepts of time and space, however, offer us infinities without the simultaneous presentation of non-space and non-time. We cannot conceive, and fundamentally we are not interested in, such curiosities. We neglect them for a variety of reasons.

The existence of ourselves is another example of an object with an implied non-being. All of us know that we are mortal, and all of us can contemplate our non-being almost at the same moment as we savour the realities of our existence.

But if man were to become immortal then self would be placed on the same footing as the unnegated concepts of space and time. But there would not be the same saving escape routes for the self. Anybody can neglect the non-negatived concept of space by pondering upon the fact that man is limited in his travelling capacities, or by not bothering to think about it at all. But man is not saved from contemplation of himself by any facts in himself, and he cannot easily stop thinking about himself, except by arranging a period of unconsciousness.

This vista of the endless, unlimited self might create a novel sort of anxiety. The antidote to it might come from immortalist man seeking to negate it by seeking an artificial death. But man would be utterly responsible then for his own destiny, whether he went on living, killed himself, or had himself killed.

A related kind of anxiety which might go hand in hand with this could be causal anxiety. In the normal lifespan causal anxiety is checked and balanced. However altruistic we may be, we are usually capable of stifling our anxieties about those of our acts whose consequences will affect our descendants. We tend to talk in rather lofty ways about building for the future, but these plans do not carry the flavour of anxiety within them.

If we are honest with ourselves, and really analyse our feelings about the future, we are probably likely to come round in the end to the view that at best we have only minimal responsibility for the future, and that our descendants and intervening accidental happenings must take their own share of the load.

It would be a different matter for the immortalists. With them the future would be much more causally significant for the obvious reason that the future would belong to them, and they would live in it. Hence they would be able to view their mistakes retrospectively, and have ample time for recriminations, and regrets.

For them pollution would not be an easily-shrugged-off threat. Conservation would take on real meaning. Words would echo for notional centuries. For these reasons and many more there would certainly develop a level of concern about actions and effects that in some cases would grow into real anxiety.

At the same time, however, we should balance this new anxiety against the pleasures of future participation. Mortal man must perform a number of laudable actions, the consequences of which he can visualize, but the fruits of which he will not see. Landscape gardening is perhaps the most obvious example of this kind of consequence-deprived sort of activity, but there are, of course, many others. They may involve slow growth or development of a biological kind, or equally slow growth in an organizational or training sense – the training of personnel for a new business, the proving of a technique over time, or the working out of a political philosophy, are all examples. The immortalist will experience all these pleasures.

To be fair we ought also to chart the disappearance of a possible source of satisfaction, the notion of death as a leveller. Death as at present seen and experienced is, as far as is known, the absolute leveller. There are, of course, certain class differentials in survival.

The rich and/or the successful can postpone their deaths by a few years, the clever and the informed possibly by a few years longer, but all eventually die. Which is another way of saying that, though we may not be equals in life, we are assuredly equals in death, even though that equality does not profit the dead.

But immortality will strip away this satisfaction. For the first time a man with no costly possessions, and little or no hope of obtaining any, will not be able to comfort himself by nihilist ruminations about bringing nothing into the world and taking nothing out. For the first time such a man will be face to face with his own inadequacies. These may or may not be permanent or irremediable, but death will not be a poultice if no other remedy can be found.

This sentiment, which is essentially a compulsion in man's thinking, brings us to contrast seeking, and the effect that immortality will have on it. There is a sense in which man's mind is a comparison-making machine, well adapted to picking out the differences between objects and arguments. As well as this capability which we could describe as immediate, the mind also has the power of imaginative contrast, it can see things both as they are and as they will be.

It is this contrast-seeking, comparison-making facility that, in a changing world full of death and decay, provides man with one of his sharpest pleasures. Beauty is of little value unless it is compared with the potential decay which lies within it. Death and disappearance, partings and meetings are the stuff of art. Without death how does Milton generate the vital emotion of grief which impels him to write *Lycidas*? What becomes of the great Shakespearean dramas that are built upon murder and usurpation?

When we contemplate a world in which death is dead as far as man is concerned, we must also gauge the effect this might have upon the aesthetic satisfactions that he gains from death's existence.

In so far as the contrast-seeking element in man's brain would still look for contrast even when death is dead, we may anticipate a much greater pressure for aesthetic satisfactions from contrast that is not death-dependent. There would presumably still be moral differentiation, a division, though not firm, between good and bad, and we may expect a concentration upon a moral art, emphasizing conduct values in social terms, and equating beauty with good.

Then, of course, there would still be cyclical and non-cyclical changes occurring environmentally: the ever-mobile sky, the seasonal variations, the dramatic fury of the elements. These would provide much material with a built-in contrast that could be instantly recognized and appreciated, and which might popularize pastoral art in various forms.

Then, we ought not to overlook the death-dependent contrasts which may be found in the existing mortality of animals, to say nothing of the probability that some people may not choose to be immortal. 'Life martyrdom', which is what we can justifiably term this choice, since it may enable procreation to continue, may well be the substance of tragic art. The lives and deaths of animals have always, of course, been part of a narrow artistic tradition. How far new pressures might broaden that tradition is difficult to say. At a guess one would predict a considerable development with a great increase in sentimentalization.

Finally we should discuss innovation. There may well be several factors involved here which may be significant in the immortalist state. Man, as distinct from woman, produces nothing which endures, and in consequence some at least of the drive to innovate must spring from his desire to create artifacts or situations that will outlast him. Immortality would deny him this motivation.

The second factor is more speculative. It is conceivable that man is unconsciously creative or innovatory because he is impotent, or feels unimportant, by comparison with the immensity of the universe. Here again if he becomes immortal he may lose that sense of inferiority which drives him on to creation. He may feel massively soothed as though the very act of becoming immortal was itself an ultimate justifying innovation.

There is one last important factor – the degree to which innovation is the product of a clash of ideas between young and old, which raises the question of how much a single-generation society actually affects the development of ideas. There is no argument about the necessity for cross-fertilization in the process of creativity. Whether we examine the process as it occurs within an individual, or within a group, there can be no doubt that the process is one of display (in the sense of ideas forced into the system and discussed or cogitated upon), recording (the combining of these ideas in new forms) and selection (the picking out of the best-fitting creations).

What is in doubt is whether the youth-versus-age combination is vital in keeping up a flow of new ideas. Flexibility of contact between creative individuals and creative groups does seem to be essential. But given the fact that all creative persons would retain their physical and intellectual powers indefinitely it would seem immaterial how continuous cross-fertilization came about, provided it came about. Thus an immortalist society which deliberately set about being creative might end up more creative by design than it might ever have been by natural accident.

Bibliography

Current Views
Harrington, Alan *The Immortalist: an approach to the engineering of man's divinity* Random House, 1969

The Engineer Intervenes
Barer, M. *et al.* 'Bone formation and resorption in normal human rib' *Clinical Orthopaedics* **52,** pp 241–47 (ed. Urist, M. R.) Pitman Medical, 1967
Fishlock, David *Man Modified* Jonathan Cape, 1969
Jowsey, J. 'Age changes in human bone' *Clinical Orthopaedics* **17,** pp 210–17 Pitman Medical, 1960
Mercer, W. and Duthie, R. B. *Orthopaedic Surgery* 6th edn Edward Arnold, 1964
Montagna, W. and Ellis, R. A. *Biology of Hair Growth* Academic Press 1958
Symposium 'Lubrication and wear in living and artificial joints' *Proc. Inst. Mech. Engineering* **181,** part 3J, 1966–67
Trueta, Joseph *Studies of the development and decay of human frame* Heinemann, 1968

A Self-maintaining Machine
Advances in Gerontological Research, Vols I and II Academic Press
Allen, J. M. (ed.) *Nature of Biological Diversity* McGraw-Hill, 1963
Birren, J. E. (ed.) *Handbook of ageing and the individual* Chicago University Press, 1959
Bourne, G. H. (ed.) *Practical aspects of ageing* Pitman, 1961
Strehler, B. L. *et al.* (ed.) *Biology of ageing* American Institute of Biology Service, 1960
Strehler, B. L. *Time Cells and Ageing* Academic Press, 1962

Telescoped Brains
Mechanisation of Thought Processes Vols I and II, HMSO, 1959

Remorseless Numbers
Jung, R. and Galtung, J. *Mankind* 2000 Allen & Unwin, 1969

Gods Themselves
Heinlein, R. A. *Methuselah's Children* Gollancz, 1963